If The Walls of My Exam Room Could Talk

Angela,

Thanks for everything!

Mark

If The Walls of My Exam Room Could Talk

Stories of Triumph

over a common
but often unrecognized
visual ailment:

Vertical Heterophoria

Debby Feinberg, O.D.
With Mark Rosner M.D. & Sherry Brantley

ISBN-13: 978-1482399790
ISBN: 1482399792

To order additional copies of _If The Walls Of My Exam Room Could Talk_ call 248-258-9000, or order online at: www.VSofM.com

Library of Congress Cataloging-in-Publication Data

Feinberg, Debby

    If the walls of my exam room could talk / Debby Feinberg -1st ed.

Cover and Cover Design by Matthew Rosner

Interior Design by Matthew Rosner and Dr. Mark Rosner

FIRST EDITION

We would like to dedicate this book to the most important people in our lives – our parents Paul, Shirley, Joel and Sarah; our children Alex and Matthew; and to our brothers and sisters and their families

ACKNOWLEDGEMENTS

So many people have helped me along the way, and I'd like to give them the recognition they deserve. First and foremost, I'd like to thank my father and colleague Dr. Paul Feinberg, who provided the time and creative working environment which allowed me to explore the solutions to help patients suffering from Vertical Heterophoria (VH). My father is also the inventor of many tools that we use on a daily basis to measure and assess prismatic requirements in our patients. I would also like to thank my mother Shirley Feinberg, who as the talented frame buyer provided patients with the frames that made them feel attractive when wearing their "eyeglass medicine". She has also been a great supporter of this work from the very beginning. I'd also like to thank my in-laws Joel and Sarah Rosner. They understood the importance and impact of this work from the very beginning and encouraged me to take the leap and open my own practice dedicated to the treatment of VH. I would also like to thank my sons Alex and Matthew, who are the loves of my life and have been very great supporters of this journey. I would like to acknowledge my colleague Dr. Morrie Dubin, and all of the staff at Vision Specialists of Michigan for the wonderful care you provide for our special patients. I would also like to thank all of the case managers, doctors and other health care providers who understood our work early on, and who helped their patients (and helped propel the work forward) by allowing us the privilege to care for them. I would also like to thank Sherry Brantley, who has enthusiastically delved into this book project. She interviewed all forty patients (and was well received by all), and turned out forty compelling stories of triumph over suffering.

Last, but not least, I'd like to thank my husband Mark, who if it weren't for his determination and efforts to move this body of knowledge forward, to collect the data and do the writing, we would not be where we are today.

MEDICAL INFORMATION IS CONSTANTLY CHANGING

The information in this book is up to date and current as of February, 2013. However, it won't be long before new discoveries are made, and our understanding of Vertical Heterophoria will expand.

To keep abreast of all of the new developments, please visit our website:

www.VSofM.com

A WORD OF CAUTION TO THE READER

The information presented in this book is based upon the training and professional experience of the author. This book was written for informational purposes. It is not intended to be used as medical advice.

Contents

Part One

Traumatic Brain Injury Stories

Part Two

Stories From Children and Teenagers

Part Three

Family Stories

Part Four

Stories Of Those Who Had Symptoms As

Children And As Adults

Part Five

Stories Of Those Who Have Dizziness And / Or Headache As Their Major Symptom(s)

Part Six

Miscellaneous Stories

Appendix

Index (by Symptoms)

FOREWORD

Dr. Arthur Rosner

While in college I was experiencing problems with my vision. I had double vision, some issues with reading and depth perception, and I was also having headaches. These were conditions I had dealt with for many years, but became more of a nuisance during my years as a medical student. To ease the task of reading, the head of ophthalmology at the University gave me a hand-held prism to hold in front of my eyes whenever I needed to, which gave me some sense of relief. A few years later, upon meeting Dr. Debby (herself a recently graduated optometrist) she saw me use the wedge of prism, and she asked me why I needed it. I explained the issues I'd been having and she asked to examine me. She found that I needed vertical prism and incorporated it into my eyeglass lenses, which made a major improvement overall for me. So out of necessity for me, and curiosity for her, I became Dr. Debby's first Vertical Heterophoria (VH) patient, and while I didn't know it yet, the first member of her Research Team.

Since the medical community is not very familiar with VH and its set of symptoms, patients and doctors tend to search in the wrong place for solutions. As an ENT (Ear/Nose/Throat) and sleep physician, I work with patients that have dizziness and headaches. People come to me with pain that they think stems from a sinus problem, or with dizziness which they think is related to the inner ear. Sometimes they are correct, but in a surprising number of cases, VH is the unsuspected and undetected culprit. In many instances I was not the first doctor to see these patients for their symptoms. Some had been to many specialists and tried multiple medications and therapies without obtaining effective reduction of symptoms. They became frustrated and depressed, as there seemed to be no answer for them.

I noticed as I was working with these patients that they had the same (or at least a similar) pattern of symptoms that I'd experienced prior to wearing Dr. Debby's prism glasses. Initially, I sent these patients to the ophthalmologist, but using the current methods and techniques to evaluate these problems, they were unable to find anything wrong with the patient's vision. I then decided to refer a few of these patients to Dr. Debby to see if she'd be able to help them as she had helped me. Those patients returned to me with astounding stories of the difference that the prism glasses had made for them. Not just minor changes, but major differences in how they were now able to function on a daily basis. We know that there will never be just one treatment that is the solution for all patients, but about 85% of the patients that I refer to Vision Specialists of Michigan are able to be helped tremendously.

As of February 2013, Vision Specialists of Michigan had seen over 7000 patients with VH, of which approximately 1000 are Traumatic Brain Injury (TBI) patients. With the use of prismatic lenses they experience on average an 80% reduction of symptoms. Some patients have been treated for over 15 years and they have maintained symptom reduction with only minor adjustments to the prism prescription during that time. It is our best estimate that at least 5% of the population may benefit from prism lenses. Five percent may sound like a small number, but it currently represents approximately 15 million Americans.

As a result of all of the patients that Vision Specialists of Michigan has been able to help over the past 17 years, the research and study that the Research Team has conducted and the tools that have been developed (such as the validated Vertical Heterophoria Symptom Questionnaire (VHSQ) and the specific methods and techniques that have been developed to diagnose and treat VH) it is clear that this is not a fad solution that will be "here today and gone tomorrow". While we understand and expect some skepticism (which is normal whenever anything new is being introduced - especially when it impacts so many medical specialties), the methods and techniques that Dr. Debby and Vision Specialists of Michigan use are based on sound, scientific principles stemming from decades of her own research and the research of others.

Dr. Debby did not begin researching this field for monetary gain. There's not a huge foundation, nor government money set aside for the study of VH or its' resolution. She feels this research is critical because when proper techniques are utilized, prism lenses can significantly alleviate or even eliminate the myriad of VH symptoms (headache, dizziness, anxiety, neck pain, reading difficulties), transforming the lives of very uncomfortable and suffering people and allowing them to live normal lives once again.

I am honored and privileged to say that I have been working in collaboration with Dr. Debby on this very compelling research since the very beginning. I have seen the good that comes from the proper treatment of VH and I am proud to do what I can to advance this work. I was pleased to have helped with the development of the VHSQ, which has proven instrumental in moving this work forward. I have lectured nationally and internationally on VH to advance the cause of bringing our research and knowledge to the medical community as well as to the public at large.

To all of you who read the amazing stories in this book, to all of the professionals in the medical community and the staff who work alongside them, to the portion of the population who may be suffering from the symptoms of Vertical Heterophoria, and to those of you who may know a family member, co-worker or friend that exhibits symptoms of VH, there is an important message I want to convey:

It is critical that this body of information be disseminated throughout the medical world and that others are taught to do this work. There were two other pioneers in the field of VH – Dr. George T. Stevens (in the 1880s) and Dr. Raymond Roy (in the 1950s) who performed groundbreaking work and yet were unable to have their knowledge widely disseminated to the medical community, preventing untold millions of people from receiving life altering care. VH impacts too many people (many severely) to allow this to happen again. It is clear that the current methods and techniques used to diagnose and treat VH are ineffective, making some people come to the conclusion that prism lenses are themselves ineffective. Dr. Debby and the Research Team at Vision Specialists of Michigan have years of in-depth study, building upon information compiled from almost two decades of their own research as well as the decades of research of others (including Stevens and Roy), and she and her clinical colleagues Dr. Paul Feinberg and Dr. Morrie Dubin have had significant quantitative success in reducing VH symptoms with prism lenses with thousands of patients over the years. They have learned and perfected the art of prescribing prisms for VH patients.

This book, combined with all of our other efforts, is our attempt to make sure that this critically important work in the area of Vertical Heterophoria and prism lenses will not get lost once again, but rather continue to grow and progress and reach the millions of people who need it.

Arthur Rosner, M.D.

   -ENT Specialist
   -VH Researcher

FOREWORD

Dr. Jennifer Doble

I learned about Vision Specialists of Michigan and the prism lenses from one of my patients. I am a physician (Physical Medicine and Rehabilitation specialist) and a large portion of my practice involves treating patients with Traumatic Brain Injury (TBI). At the time, my hospital and my medical practice were converting to computerized medical records and I'd begun having horrible headaches. I was also experiencing fatigue and dizziness. My patient informed me that she'd been referred to a special optometrist, and was given a new prescription for her eyeglasses which gave her improvement not only with her vision, but with other symptoms she'd been having - symptoms that were similar to what I'd been experiencing personally. Curious, I asked more questions and she began to tell me about her prism glasses and all the differences they were able to make for her.

During this time, I had been looking for a new optometrist for myself, and after hearing this patient's progress directly from her, I thought it would be a good idea for me to be evaluated by Dr. Feinberg.

During my first eye exam, I learned something from Dr. Feinberg that made perfect sense to me. An ophthalmologist had provided me with glasses which had a prism lens for one eye, but not the other. Dr. Feinberg explained to me that if you have Vertical 4Heterophoria (VH) you can't treat just one eye - you have to treat and take care of both since VH is a condition that affects both eyes. With the prism glasses she prescribed, I was able to tell a difference right away. To this day, my eyes are working better together and they feel more relaxed, and my headaches are much less intense and I have them less often. I have definitely experienced dramatic improvement in my symptoms.

During my eye examination, Dr. Feinberg shared with me the work she was doing with VH, and I thought it sounded like something that would be helpful for my head injury patients. Up until then, I had been referring my patients to neuroophthalmologists (eye surgeons that specialize in finding and treating eye movement or vision problems originating from a neurological problem). Some were treated with medication and physical therapy, but it didn't alleviate the symptoms of headache, dizziness and fatigue they had been experiencing.

The first few patients I sent to Dr. Feinberg came back with good results. Their dizziness and headaches had subsided, they were no longer fatigued, and they had stopped experiencing the eye strain. I was able to take them off of medications. They reported to me that they could clearly see and read the newspaper and the computer screen without any strain, and that they actually felt comfortable when doing so. The impact that the prism glasses were able to make was significant, so I began to refer more patients to her.

For patients that have experienced a TBI, a typical day can involve dealing with many different issues, including fatigue, headaches, cognitive impairment, anxiety, and irritability. Some are trying to get back to work, and may be emotionally insecure as to whether or not they'll ever be able to function normally again. The prism glasses give patients visual clarity so that they're not only visually focused but cognitively focused as well. They feel much less dizziness and fatigue. They no longer feel as if they're in a constant visual and cognitive fog. This allows their self-confidence and emotional outlook to improve as well.

There are many people who are suffering from the various symptoms of VH who are being told that there's nothing that can be done for them except to prescribe drugs. For many of them, the prism glasses can be a fabulous, non-chemical solution. It is not an invasive, expensive surgery. It's simply a specialized pair of lenses that act as a "visual orthotic" (not unlike how a heel lift works for a person with a leg length discrepancy). It's probably one of the best medical improvements we have had to help treat brain injury patients in decades. Because of the commitment and passion that Dr. Feinberg has in working in this area, we're now able to provide her optical treatment techniques to many patients, using this simple yet powerful solution.

It is my sincere hope that neuroophthalmologists, optometrists, and others in the health care field read the stories within the pages of this book, and realize the benefit of prism glasses. These stories are in the words of the patients and represent their experiences, detailing the various symptoms that they'd suffered prior to finding out about VH, and how receiving a correct prism prescription for their glasses made a world of difference. I'm well aware that there will be the naysayers, and those that find it hard to believe that all of these improvements can happen with just a pair of prism glasses. However, I would hope that once the healthcare providers are exposed to actual patients who have experienced these changes and really hear the difference it has made in their lives, they too will become advocates.

I support Dr. Feinberg in developing a training program for other optometrists, and look forward to a time when all patients with TBI will have access to this treatment option.

Jennifer Doble, M.D.

   -Physical Medicine and Rehabilitation physician
   -TBI Specialist
   -VH Researcher

INTRODUCTION
Dr. Debby Feinberg

I have listened to over 7000 patients in 17 years tell their stories that up until now were not understood by their doctors. My patients felt frustrated, misunderstood, not believed, and worst of all felt that there was no relief for their suffering.

These patients were called crazy, psychogenic and hypochondriacal. They were told that they must be making it up. They looked fine, but didn't feel fine. Sometimes they did not want to continue living. Their symptoms were real, and their lives were becoming more limited with each passing day, month and year. Their strategies for survival included reducing their exposure to stimulating environments, dimming the lights in their homes, avoiding group gatherings, avoiding highway driving, and sometimes abandoning driving altogether. Ultimately, they found it more and more difficult to live the life that they wanted to live, and work in the work place that they wanted to be in. Getting through each day was becoming a difficult chore. A previously pleasurable activity like going to the mailbox or taking the dog for a walk became an overwhelming task. They found themselves choosing the safety of their home rather than venturing out where they might get in an accident or have trouble getting home safely. As the search for answers came up short, even the people themselves began to doubt the realness of their own symptoms. Maybe it was all in their head? Maybe they were never going to get better?

Well, this group of people refused to give up. They were determined and kept searching for answers to find relief from their debilitating symptoms of headaches, dizziness, anxiety, nausea, imbalance with walking, light sensitivity, neck pain, and reading challenges.

Finally (sometimes after many years of suffering) they started to find their way to our office. Sometimes it was a phone call from a friend or relative who had received relief, sometimes it was a referral from a doctor, and sometimes it was from a forum on the internet. A number of people would search their symptoms on the internet and up popped the office website. They would fill out the online questionnaire and one of the doctors or staff members would call them to let them know that they were most likely suffering from a poorly understood and infrequently recognized vision condition that could be successfully treated with custom glasses containing realigning prisms. It was often quite a shock for the patient to learn that a vision problem might be at the root of all of their symptoms, and that a pair of special glasses might offer them relief. How could the answer be so simple?

This book will tell the story of the serendipitous way in which the diagnosis and treatment of Vertical Heterophoria (VH) came to be discovered, as well as a description of VH for patients and for doctors. The majority of the book will be used to relate the stories of 40 patients who are now living their lives again more fully, with marked reduction or even elimination of their symptoms.

If the walls of my exam room could talk, this book would not be needed. You would have already heard these stories, as would have the medical community, and VH would be an easily identifiable and treatable condition. By giving a voice to the walls of my exam room, I hope to bring attention to this condition so that everyone (patients and doctors alike) can recognize it, understand it, and obtain successful treatment for it.

This book has been written so that my patients' stories will finally be heard - of their terrible suffering with VH, and the seemingly miraculous improvement with prismatic lenses. These are important stories, and they need to be told. For those people who have yet to find the answer to their symptoms, my prayer is that they will read this book and learn that there is hope and help for them, too!

Debby Feinberg, O.D.

-Neurovisual Optometrist
-VH Researcher

How To Use This Book

It is the aim of this book to explain, through patient stories and explanatory documents, what VH is and how it affects people. It is hoped that it will be used to help individuals identify that they or a loved one or friend might be suffering from VH and need the help of a Neurovisual optometrist. It is also hoped that this book will be utilized by the medical community to help them understand the full ramifications of VH, and to aid in the identification of their patients who might have VH and benefit from a Neurovisual evaluation.

STORIES

This book is a compilation of stories of patients who have been diagnosed and treated for Vertical Heterophoria (VH). Reading all of the stories will impart to the reader the many and varied combinations of symptoms a patient can experience due to VH. However, there are some major themes, and the book has been arranged to highlight them:

Part One: Traumatic Brain Injury Stories

The most common cause of VH is congenital (i.e. – you are born with it). The symmetry of the shape of your face and the location of your eye sockets, and the symmetry between the eye muscles and their innervation is determined by the time you are born. These people usually become symptomatic with VH by the age of 40, though there are some who become symptomatic at an earlier age, some as early as 4 years old.

The second most common cause of VH is Acquired Brain Injury (ABI), of which Traumatic Brain Injury (TBI) is by far the most frequent reason. TBI's most often occur from Motor Vehicle Accidents (MVA's), but can also be caused by sports injuries (e.g. - football, soccer, hockey, lacrosse, skiing), and combat injuries (explosions from bombs and IED's). Our clinic sees a large number of these patients. It is currently estimated that half of all TBI patients who experience prolonged post-concussive symptoms can be helped with glasses with prismatic lenses.

Part Two: Stories From Children and Teenagers

While people with VH usually become symptomatic around the age of 40, it is not uncommon to have younger people be afflicted with VH. It is important that those who provide medical and psychological and reading and learning services to children become familiar with the symptoms associate with VH, so that they can refer those who need it for a Neurovisual assessment.

Part Three: Family Stories

Have you ever noticed how members of the same family share many facial characteristics (i.e. - they all look like each other)? The shape and symmetry of your face is very much influenced by your heredity (i.e. – your family genetics), so it is not surprising that VH also "runs in families". If one member of the family has VH, it is almost certain that a sibling, parent, child, aunt, uncle or cousin will also have VH.

Part Four: Stories of Those Who Had Symptoms as Children and as Adults

Many adults had their initial VH symptoms begin as children, and if they could have been identified and treated at that point, many years of discomfort and disability could have been avoided. Those who provide care for children must become familiar with the set of symptoms that constitutes VH.

Part Five: Stories of Those Who Have Dizziness and / or Headache as Their Major Symptom(s)

The majority of VH patients have either headache or dizziness (or both) as one of their major symptoms. These patients have routinely been seen by multiple specialists, and tried many different medications and treatments and yet still are suffering from their headache / dizziness. These are the most challenging and frustrating patients that the doctors see, because no matter how hard the doctor tries, the patient just never seems to get better.

Part Six: Miscellaneous Stories

Stories that don't conveniently fit into the other categories are found in this section.

APPENDIX

There are four items within the Appendix – two questionnaires and two articles. The questionnaires are the Adult VHSQ (Vertical Heterophoria Symptom Questionnaire) and the Pediatric VHSQ. These survey instruments have been developed to help identify those who might be suffering from VH. Feel free to make a copy of the questionnaires and use them yourself, or give them to a friend or loved one you suspect might have VH. Using the scoring mechanism, find out if they have a score of $\geq$ 15. If they do, consultation with a Neurovisual optometrist is recommended.

The two articles explain how VH makes you sick (the pathophysiology). The first article is written for everyone; the second article is directed at medical professionals.

INDEX

In this book, the Index has been used to allow for identification of stories by specific symptom. If the patient had significant difficulties with a certain symptom, it is referenced in the Index.

Our "Discovery" of Vertical Heterophoria

It was 1985, and I was on a double-date with the man who eventually became my husband (Mark) and his brother (Arthur) and his soon-to-be wife. We were driving along when I noticed he was holding a large hand-held prism up to one of his eyes. Being an optometrist, I recognized what it was and asked him what he was doing with it. He explained that he had been having eye strain issues, and had seen the chief of Ophthalmology at his medical school. He had a thorough eye exam, yet nothing was found amiss. Arthur maintained that there must be something wrong, as he could feel the strain, and the doctor gave him the hand-held prism, with the instructions to exercise his eyes with it to see if he could reduce the feelings of strain. "So, has it helped?" I asked. "Not much" was his reply. So I suggested that he come in for an eye exam, and if he really needed a prismatic correction, I could make it part of his prescription in his lenses and he could wear it fulltime. It turned out he needed vertical prismatic correction, and Arthur became my first Vertical Heterophoria (VH) patient.

Unbeknownst to me, Arthur had other symptoms that the prism lenses had corrected. Reading was challenging, and he had difficulty with depth perception. He was a practicing ENT physician, and as he cared for his patients, he realized that many of them who were suffering with dizziness and headache did not have a problem with their inner ear (as their inner ear testing had been normal). As he listened more closely to their histories, it dawned on him that they were having symptoms similar to what he had experienced because of his VH. Could it be that they had an eye alignment problem, too? He then began to refer them to their eye care providers, but a funny thing happened. They all came back saying that their evaluations had all been normal – no visual problems or misalignments. This just didn't make sense to Arthur – they had the same symptoms after all, how could this be?

One day in 1995 I got a call from Arthur. "Debby, I want to send you some of my dizzy patients." "Why would you want to do that?" I said. "I'm an optometrist – I take care of healthy people with blurry vision. I've never taken care of dizzy people." Then Arthur said, "You took care of me, and I got better with prism lenses. These patients sound a lot like me, and I think you can help them." "OK," I said, "I'll see just a couple, and see what I can do."

He initially sent me two sisters. They shuffled in using canes to help with their balance, and they had sick-bags, in case they needed to vomit. And he thinks I can help these people? I was beginning to think that this was strange, but they were here, so I examined them. It turned out that they both indeed did have vertical misalignment, and both felt markedly better with prismatic lenses.

This was almost unbelievable! I had never been trained in optometry school about this. We knew about vertical misalignment, but for the most part we were discouraged from even taking the measurements – they were hard to interpret, and they were difficult to use to make adjustments to the lens prescription. If it wasn't for my dad *insisting* that I take those measurements when I was a new graduate, I would never have found the vertical misalignment in Arthur or these two sisters.

And the symptoms – while we might have taught that eye misalignment could cause eye pain (asthenopia) and maybe headache and some challenges reading, we had never been taught that it could cause:

Pain symptoms: migraines, face pain

Vestibular symptoms: dizziness, vertigo, motion sickness (even as a child), nausea, anorexia, drifting while walking, problems with balance and coordination, falling

Psychiatric symptoms: anxiety, agoraphobia, panic attacks, suicidal ideation, overwhelmed in crowds or malls

Neck pain: due to head tilt

Visual symptoms: shadowed vision, difficulty being fit with glasses

Reading symptoms: visual hallucination of letters / words moving on the page, dyslexia, skipping lines, difficulty with comprehension

And here I was helping all of these patients with medical problems with prismatic lenses!

I was only working part time (since my children were young at the time), but by 2004 I had seen 500 VH patients. Arthur and I had by then developed a questionnaire to help identify who might have VH (which has since been validated – the VHSQ (Vertical Heterophoria Symptom Questionnaire)). We presented this information at the AAO-HNS (American Academy of Otolaryngologists – Head and Neck Surgeons) Annual Meeting in 2005, and it was well received.

About this time, a patient who had been injured in a car accident came in for treatment of VH symptoms, and they did well. The next thing I know, I'm getting a call from the patient's PM&R (Physical Medicine and Rehabilitation) doctor, wanting to know more about what I was doing. Her patient had been through all kinds of treatments but had never responded like this – she was so much better! The more we talked, the more it became apparent that this doctor also had VH symptoms from childhood. She came and was evaluated as a patient, she did have VH, and she responded beautifully to prismatic lenses. These experiences led her to realize that VH symptoms are almost the same as "post-concussive symptoms", and that almost all of her brain injured patients had these symptoms (she had a practice that specialized in brain injury). Could it be that brain injury patients had VH, and if so, could they be helped with prismatic lenses?

The PM&R doctor is Jennifer Doble, and the answer is appearing to be that TBI patients do have VH, and the symptoms are markedly reduced with prismatic lenses. We have currently evaluated and treated over 1000 brain injury patients with very positive results.

Review of the literature demonstrates that VH was initially identified by Dr. George T. Stevens, an ophthalmologist, in 1887. He tried treating it with prism, but he used large amounts and was unsuccessful, so he treated it surgically with good results, but no one has been able to reproduce his work. The next person to significantly discuss VH was Dr. Raymond Roy, an optometrist who wrote 11 articles describing his findings in the 1950s and 1960s. He would patch an eye for 6 days in order to determine what misalignment existed. This was not well received by his patients, and other eye care providers did not pick up on his techniques. VH has been minimally described in the optometry texts (Borish), and more extensively described in the ophthalmology tome edited by Duke-Elder. The problem that has plagued identifying and researching VH is that the vertical measurements are not very accurate, particularly in very small amounts. Our data demonstrates that these measurements are actually very flawed, and this caused us to develop other techniques to identify vertical misalignment that were not tied to these measurements. This, and using very small increments of prism, have allowed us to finally be able to identify and care for this suffering population of people.

To date, my office colleagues and I have seen over 7,000 of these patients. Our best estimate is that VH affects 5-10% of the human population. I get e-mails and calls every day from around the world asking for help, which makes me believe that our estimates are correct. It is clear that this information needs to be disseminated broadly, so that those who are suffering from this condition can be identified and treated. We have a long way to go on that mission, and this book is part of that effort.

It appears that our "discovery" of VH was really a "re-discovery". It is our hope that "the third time is the charm," and that this time we are successful in getting information about VH into the hands of the professionals that can help patients with this condition, as well as into the hands of the average person so they can "self-identify" themselves and get the help they need.

It is clear to me that the history of VH is still being written, and I am looking forward to the next chapters!

Debby Feinberg, O.D.

-Neurovisual Optometrist

-VH Researcher

Part One

Traumatic Brain Injury Stories

I Came Using My Walker, Left Walking On My Own

By Carl Fancil

Driving home late one night, after babysitting my grandchildren, I had no idea I would be involved in a major car accident. I was heading on I-275, just outside of Detroit, preparing to take the Ford Rd. exit from the freeway, when suddenly I was rear-ended by a vehicle which had been traveling at a very high speed. In a matter of mere seconds, my vehicle flipped three times before resting on its' wheels. My air bags deployed, and my laptop went flying through my sunroof, skidding along the icy pavement as smoothly as an Olympic ice skater. It was February 14, 2010, and this terrible accident changed my life from that day on.

Miraculously, I was able to walk away from the accident, and while still in shock, was not able to discern any major damage beyond the bumps and bruises that being in such an accident would incur. A passer-by stopped to offer assistance prior to the police and ambulance being called, and she too, was surprised I was unscathed. She offered me a ride, as my vehicle was totaled.

I took a trip to the emergency room to ensure that no internal injuries had occurred, and was sent home with instructions to follow up with my family physician. During that follow up visit, I told my doctor about getting headaches and dizziness, and he immediately said that I'd suffered a concussion. I was admitted to a local hospital for a few days to have a head CT (among other tests) and to be observed. At this time, it was clear that I was beginning to experience the physical symptoms of a brain injury as a result of the car accident.

The headaches were one of the first of many symptoms. But this wasn't just your 'average headache.' It was a constant throbbing pain, felt just behind my eyes and across my forehead, that wasn't alleviated or eliminated by headache medication. It was a pain that was now a constant companion.

As the weeks and months passed by, my symptoms increased. Throughout the day I would feel faint and dizzy. I began to experience vertigo, and was no longer able to drive. In addition to those symptoms, I began falling a lot and therefore had to use a cane, which eventually gave way to my needing to use a walker. The combination of these symptoms led to my having anxiety issues. Not knowing when I would feel dizzy or when I might be hurt in a slip and fall became of great concern to me.

As time progressed, I was seeing a host of different doctors and specialists, attempting to pinpoint what was wrong with me and to see what could be done to get my life back on track. One of the specialists, who came to me as a referral, discovered that I'd suffered a right-lobe brain injury as a result of the accident.

As a retired police officer, after having had 30 years on the job, it was very challenging (to say the least) to now have to experience life in such a debilitating and limiting way. My wife and I loved to travel and this was the time we'd envisioned we'd be able to do so with pleasure. But now, just looking down at the sidewalk literally made me sick. I'd become dizzy and prone to walking unsteadily. Seven and a half months after the accident, I was still seeing specialists and having tests run. I was getting depressed and unable to focus clearly. As a police officer, I'd experienced many circumstances when people had felt hopeless with nowhere to turn;

when they felt that no life at all would be better than the one they were experiencing, but I'd never imagined that I too, would come to feel that way.

By the time I received the referral to see Dr. Debby Feinberg, it'd been a year after the accident, and I was seeing a number of different doctors for the range of symptoms that I was experiencing. When I received the referral, I was willing to try anything for even a little relief. But going to my appointment with her that day provided me with so much more than just a 'little relief!'

Prior to becoming a patient of Dr. Debby's, all of my other recovery was slow. This is not to negate what the other specialists were doing for me, but in order to fix what is wrong, you have to know where to look. Dr. Debby seemed to have a knack for that. Before going to her, and with my using a walker, everything in my life was turned upside-down. I had a real problem with motivation. All I wanted to do was sleep all the time. Sometimes, my own voice vibrated pain within my inner ear. I was no longer able to engage in my hobbies such as sand-blasting-glass-shaping, wood carving or anything. I now had no drive, motivation or inclination to even attempt to do any of those things and besides, my eyesight and my other symptoms did not allow me to.

My vision was so bad that I'd look at something on a wall, and see a second one—a dual image. The second one was to the right and dropped down a bit from the original image, but it was just as clear as if it were actually there, proving I could no longer trust my own eyesight.

My wife had to drive me to my appointment at Dr. Debby's' office. From that very first appointment, it was clear she was of a different breed of eye doctor. I was there for three hours for my first visit. It was the best three hours I'd ever spent, because I'd gone there using a walker, but left walking out on my own, without any assistance! I know it sounds hard to believe, but it's true. My wife was astounded and I was elated. Dr. Debby had me wear a pair of the prism test glasses and then took me outside to walk in them. I was walking confidently and steadily, which I hadn't been able to do in a year. I saw a penny lying on the ground and instinctively reached down to pick it up. I was able to do so without losing my balance, falling, or even getting dizzy. And this was just my first appointment with her! Even today for me, it is hard to believe that something as simple as a pair of eyeglasses could make such a world of difference in my life.

I haven't told too many people this, but before I went to Dr. Feinberg I was feeling down, depressed, and I just wasn't happy. I felt like putting an end to everything. Without the prism glasses, I don't know if I would've made it through. All that I valued no longer mattered. Everything centered upon my vision. The prism glasses helped me deal with what was going on and allowed me to get back on the right footing. The glasses eliminated the headache, which had been a constant throbbing for me. Before the glasses, everything else in my life took a backseat. Having the glasses changed ALL of that. Having Dr. Debby treat me was the main thing that turned me around and allowed me to be able to really see the light at the end of the tunnel. It had an uplifting, profound effect on me. I couldn't believe the difference - it was like going to a faith-healer! She has a definite people-skill that only magnifies the talent she has in working with your vision.

Before the prism glasses, my will to live was slowly ebbing away. After the glasses, my physical therapy exercises completely changed. I was walking unassisted, and the icing on the cake was when I was able to be certified to drive again.

The important thing for me is to let others know of the work Dr. Debby and her associates are doing, and the many patients they've been able to help. Especially those that have been told there is no help for them. It's sad when some people can't go back to work, are no longer able to drive, or are using canes and walkers because they have vertigo or are prone to dizziness and falling, when the simple solution may be to just have their vision properly checked, and if needed, getting a pair of prism glasses. She has not only helped me, but family members and others that I've referred to her. I tell others: If you are experiencing dizziness, migraines, having sensitivity to light or vertigo, you would do yourself a favor to check out her website and complete the survey. Going to see Dr. Debby could mean a life-altering change for you.

Immediately, I Stood Taller, No More Anxiety, No More Cane!

By Wanda A.   *Story 2*

In 2009, as a result of having tripped on an uneven portion of a sidewalk, I fell, which landed me on my hands and knees, causing only a slight jarring of my head and neck. I wasn't aware of any major damage initially. After getting up and dusting myself off a bit, I continued on with my activities for the day.

However, when I got to my office I felt dizzy, light-headed, nauseous and anxious, but I simply thought these were all just initial reactions to having taken a tumble. A trip to the emergency room did not yield anything major and I was sent home with some pain pills. I felt better for short periods of time, but the dizziness, nausea and anxiety would reemerge. A subsequent visit to the emergency room revealed a slight crack to the bone in my knee, but nothing else.

I had a lot of things going on in my life at the time. It was the last month of Grad School for me, as well as my last month of teaching before summer recess, and my son was going to be graduating from high school within a few short weeks. As my symptoms persisted, I assumed I was exhausted with everything that I was doing, and that perhaps I was simply becoming anxious and feeling overwhelmed with all of my upcoming activities.

When it came time for my son's graduation day, I felt terribly ill. I was nauseous, light-headed and began to have a tingling that ran down my neck to my back. I couldn't understand why I was feeling this way. The high school ceremony was to be held at

Michigan State University and I just couldn't go with the way I was feeling.

At this point I had begun to lose weight dramatically. I noticed that I felt nauseous and anxious on a daily basis. I had never felt like that before. Just the thought of going places would cause a major anxiousness within me, and when I'd ride in the car I had motion sickness that was unbearable.

I hadn't a clue what was wrong with me, and eventually wound up seeing different specialists including a gastroenterologist, endocrinologist, and a cardiologist. I also saw a neurologist for the headaches I was having, but none of these avenues were able to provide a solution for me. I saw a chiropractor in order to have adjustment work done, but it would only last for a few days, after which my aches and pains would always return, and I'd have to start all over again with treatments.

Due to all of my symptoms, I wound up having to work from home for a period of time. When I was able to return to work, initially I was only able to do so on a part-time basis.

One day, while preparing to go to work, I bent over slightly and noticed a sharp pain in my shoulder blades. The next thing I knew I had fainted and ended up on the floor! This led to another visit to the emergency room, and this time they discovered that I had low blood pressure.

All of my other symptoms were still present - the headaches, dizziness, neck, shoulder and back pain, and nausea. Unable to discern when or if I'd have another fainting spell, I was no longer comfortable enough to drive to work. I arranged to get dropped off and picked up afterwards. By the end of the spring semester, I had to take time off from work again because standing to teach in front of the class would cause me to become dizzy for no apparent reason, and it was too difficult for me to work through it. The dizziness would make my neck and back muscles tighten up, causing undue stress and pain in those areas.

A few months off from work eased my symptoms somewhat, and I was able to return to work the following year. Unfortunately, shortly thereafter I wound up falling again, this time hitting my head. I had just attended an event that had taken place in a very large room. There were lots of people at this event, many individual conversations were taking place, and it was much more activity than I'd experienced for quite some time. I felt overwhelmed and sat from time to time to relax. When I left, I was walking across the campus and it was a really nice day with the sun shining brightly down. I squinted my eyes to block out the searing sun and I remember wishing I'd brought my sunglasses along. Suddenly, I felt myself falling forward and realized I wasn't going to be able to break my fall. My head crashed unprotected, directly onto the pavement.

The fall this time resulted in my being unable to work for nearly a year. I was out from September 2010 through August 2011. My dizzy spells worsened, and my journey to various specialists in the health care field continued. Since the problem seemed to stem from my being unable to balance, I sought an ENT (Ear Nose & Throat) specialist to determine if perhaps there was an inner ear issue that had not been addressed. I had been placed on numerous medications from various specialists throughout this entire ordeal, to help alleviate my symptoms and function properly. Valium would help at times with the dizziness, but even that would only last a few hours.

The neurologist I had been seeing recommended me to a new specialist that was well-known for his techniques with migraines.

The new specialist told me that all of the obvious headache treatments had been tried without success, and he suggested that I go to an internationally renowned headache clinic for two weeks, where they would conduct extensive testing while using different medications and therapies to determine the cause of my migraines. I went, and while there I tried to talk with them about my other symptoms as well, but they didn't take an active interest in those issues at all. I would complain about the constant neck and back pain, my nausea and my dizziness, but they'd only ask at what level of pain my headache was. I felt alone in my battle to regain my full health.

A few days before I was to be released from the headache clinic, my hospital roommate (who had also been suffering from symptoms that were similar to mine) advised me she'd been given a recommendation to an eye specialist and was told she might have a condition called Vertical Heterophoria (VH). Neither of us had heard that term before, but I had my laptop with me and decided to look it up. I was shocked at what I discovered. Many of the symptoms of VH were exactly what I'd been experiencing! The more I read it, the more I thought: *This is describing me.* My hospital roommate was released a few days before I was scheduled to go home. Before I left the headache clinic, I had a spinal tap done, which caused a spinal headache that resulted in my having to get a blood patch. With the various medications they placed me on, I simply felt drugged throughout most of the day.

I was at the point of thinking: *"Something's gotta give here."* By now, I was walking with a cane, felt fatigued a lot, felt myself lean towards one side, and I continued to lose my balance when walking. I would also have motion sickness when riding in the back of the car, and would get really tired and lose my place a lot when reading.

My doctors began to tell me that I didn't need to use a cane - that I should 'just walk,' and that it was time for me to return to work. I would tell them I had to sit down just to rest at times, that I wasn't using a cane just to have it, and that after my two bad falls resulting in so many injuries I simply did not feel comfortable at all without it. Even now I get upset that I was told to 'just walk.'

While the doctors at the headache clinic hadn't given me the same recommendation for Vision Specialists as my hospital roommate had been given, after about a month I decided to E-mail my roommate to learn the results of her consultation.

She E-mailed me back immediately and told me she'd been prescribed a pair of prism glasses, and that they'd worked so well for her that she was not experiencing any headaches and was no longer on headache medication! She concluded by saying that she felt wonderful. She encouraged me to take the on-line questionnaire first, and told me if I felt I might be a candidate for their services, to contact Vision Specialists and make an appointment for myself. I was eager to go on-line and complete the survey. When I did, I couldn't believe it. Many of the questions described just what I'd been complaining about to all of my specialists! A few days after taking the survey, Dr. Debby called me directly and advised that after reviewing my information she thought it might be useful for me to come for an evaluation.

At my doctor's appointment the very next day, I mentioned to him the information I'd discovered about Vision Specialists, advised him that I'd like to make an appointment with them, and asked him what his feelings were on that. He said he thought that was a good idea, as there wasn't going to be any type of invasive procedure and it wouldn't hurt to try it. In addition, he was aware of Dr. Debby Feinberg's work, which I found comforting. He told me he'd make the referral for an evaluation, which was good because

I'd already made up my mind I was going after checking out the website and talking with Dr. Debby.

My husband accompanied me to my initial appointment. After I was fit with a pair of the prism test glasses, my results were immediate (within 20-30 minutes). My husband said to Dr. Debby: "I haven't seen her shoulders relax like that in two years." It felt so unreal. I didn't feel anxious, I stood taller, and I was able to get rid of my cane! In fact it felt so miraculous to me that I did not want to leave without having my own pair right then and there! Even though that was not possible, Dr. Debby sympathized with me, and allowed me to leave with a pair of the prism test glasses. I had immediate relief from my symptoms and that was all that mattered.

Since I've had my prism glasses, I no longer get motion sickness when riding in the car. I've weaned off of many of the medications that I'd been taking. I no longer get tired when reading. My vision is still changing, but there have been many marked, definite improvements. Even family members have remarked on the differences they've been able to see with me. One of them said to me: "Wow, you are able to move around uninhibited, you're more animated and you seem so full of life."

A lot more people need to hear about the work that Vision Specialists does and how they, too, may be able to personally benefit from these services. I told the faculty members that I work with all about Vertical Heterophoria and encouraged them to go on-line to the website, so that they could familiarize themselves with the symptoms of VH so that they might be able to recognize it in their patients and get them help.

My quest had taken me to see a neurologist, acupuncturist, chiropractor, cranial-sacral therapist, holistic healer, naturopath - anything I could try without hurting myself. Hopefully after reviewing Vision Specialists' website and perhaps submitting the survey, you can avoid having to take a similar protracted and expensive journey.

These prism glasses have been a life-saver for me. I feel better more and more each day. It's simply been amazing. Dr. Debby has been the first doctor that seemed to truly understand what I was going through and to relate how those issues impacted me on a daily basis. She's extremely genuine and sincere with everything she does with her patients.

VH Causes Symptoms That Healthcare Professionals Need To Know About

By Bryan Rush (with J. Smith, OT)   *Story 3*

This story is being told by Bryan Rush, a patient that eventually received a pair of prism glasses, and J. Smith, his Occupational Therapist, who was instrumental in assisting him in doing so.

J. Smith: In my field (Occupational Therapy) we look at how a person functions, and a person's vision has a great impact on how they function on a daily basis. Typically a person has their vision checked to simply determine how clearly they are able to see. As a rule, we're not trained to look that closely for those fine little differences that may be occurring in the eyes. Since vision isn't our area of expertise, it's an area that isn't really being assessed during the time we're working with patients. Initially when meeting Bryan, he'd complained about his eyes and we'd arranged for him to be evaluated by a typical Optometrist, and by typical I simply mean an Optometrist that does the usual everyday evaluations but who isn't aware of Vertical Heterophoria. The prescription glasses that Bryan was given weren't right for him, and he refused to wear them.

Bryan: I was experiencing double vision. I was already wearing glasses but they weren't effective for me and I couldn't see clearly through them. As a result

I simply chose not to wear them. I do needlepoint and I couldn't see well enough to put the thread through the needle. For that part of the task I would use a needle threader. I mentioned this to Joan, the Occupational Therapist that was working with me, and she took a picture of my eyes to see if she was able to notice any slight differences between them.

J. Smith: I began doing a test to see if my clients' eyes are aligned symmetrically by taking a look at the glint in their eyes. Normally the glint should be in the same place in each eye, but sometimes when looking at the patient, it's not obvious when the glints are not symmetrical. Therefore, I take a photo of the eyes - I call this test the *'Birthday Candle Test.'* I turn out the lights in the room, and I have a lit birthday candle, and I have the person hold it as if they are about to blow out the candle. It accentuates the glint in the person's eyes. I then take their picture which I use as the still-photo to determine where the glints are in the eyes to see if they are misaligned or not.

I noticed with Bryan, when I was approaching him, sometimes he'd tilt his head back, which is an indication that he may have difficulty with perceiving distance.

Bryan: I wasn't able to see well at all, and sometimes, in order to know which direction to go or where to seat myself in a session room, I adopted a method of counting the ceiling tiles to help direct me. Looking to the right would give me a feeling of disillusionment and cause anxiety, and I found

54

looking up at the ceiling would have a calming effect on me. I'd experienced a closed-head injury 10 years ago, which is when I began having problems with my vision, started feeling dizzy and was getting really confused on a daily basis.

J. Smith: Bryan tried to tell me in the beginning of our sessions that his eyes weren't working properly and to please get him some more glasses. I contacted his doctor and relayed that he needed different glasses, yet Bryan's doctor assured me that his eyes were fine. But Bryan was adamant that he needed glasses and through my persistence, I was finally able to get another pair for him.

Bryan: But that didn't solve my problem. When I wore them, I began having constant feelings of being nauseated and having headaches. I experienced a kind of double vision where people and objects seemed to look hazy to me. When two or more people stood closely, their faces seemed to merge together, and this caused even more confusion and frustration for me.

J. Smith: At first we didn't correlate this with his vision because of the other symptoms he was complaining about. We focused on his feelings of having headaches and being nauseated, trying to determine what was causing those symptoms in an effort to relieve them.

At the time, I didn't know about Vision Specialists or the work they do in the area of prism glasses, and to me, there was nothing that gave me any indication that physically Bryan's eyes weren't working in conjunction with each other. I was aware of the *'Birthday Candle Test'* that I was developing, but I knew nothing of the relationship of eye misalignment to Vertical Heterophoria.

I first found out about Dr. Debby and Vision Specialists of Michigan while working with a client who was experiencing problems with her eyesight. She'd been told by a top university clinic that there was nothing wrong with her eyes and that she just needed to pay closer attention to things and she'd be fine. This patient had explained some symptoms in her initial intake interview that we had no idea about: feeling anxious when in crowds, feelings of unsteadiness when walking, and becoming withdrawn from society and from life in general. It just so happens that the Case Manager was familiar with the research that Dr. Debby and her staff at Vision Specialists had refined in the area of prism glasses, and she recommended that the patient make an appointment there. After learning of the referral, I wanted to know more about what Vision Specialists does to see if any of my patients that could benefit from their services. In my research I learned about all of the symptoms Vertical Heterophoria can cause - symptoms that other professionals in the health care fields need to be made aware of. As I learned more about Vertical Heterophoria and what Vision Specialists was doing for these patients it dawned on me that perhaps Bryan could be helped by them as well.

Bryan: When I was first recommended to Vision Specialists and told about the work they do with helping people with their vision as well as the other symptoms they were having, I was really excited. I felt like that character in *"The Blues Brothers"* when he says: 'I can see the light!' I thought to myself: 'For the first time in close to ten years, I'm going to be able to see the light.' When I told people I was going to the eye doctor, they said: "You're going to see an eye doctor?" I'd reply: "No, not going to see 'an' eye-doctor, I'm going to THE eye doctor, the one that really works and really counts in making a difference!"

The appointment itself was a great experience. I was so excited about the prospect of finally getting my eyes taken care of that I didn't have any built-up anxiety. The staff went out of their way to make sure I felt comfortable and at ease. It was very calming and relaxing. Unlike other places that I'd gone to, Vision Specialists didn't make me feel as if I were being judged for my difficulties and the issues I was experiencing. Dr. Debby asked me about everything that I was having problems with, and she sat and listened to me explain it all to her. It was a rewarding experience for me.

After my appointment, I was even more thrilled. I stepped outside wearing my prism test glasses and I could see the clouds! Before the prism glasses, they only appeared as one big lump for me. Now, I could see their individual geometric shapes, and I was able to clearly see the colors that the sun made in reflecting from them. It was such a beautiful sight for me! It was like the difference between night and day. I could see the specific dimensions of my surroundings. The colors of the trees and colors in general were more alive. Before, I couldn't differentiate between dark blues, reds and browns. They all just seemed to run together. Now I could see them in their own right. I tell you, when I first stepped outside from the clinic wearing the prism test glasses, I didn't want to go back inside! It really was as if I'd been blind for 10 years. I used to see everything as broad, blurry objects. With the prism glasses I could now see things as if through a microscope. Everything was tuned in to its' finite details, clear and concise.

The first major improvement for me was being able to distinguish the digits on the phone, which allowed me to clearly see the different extension numbers. I was working as a volunteer receptionist, and before getting my prism glasses, it was a nightmare for me because I just couldn't see the numbers clearly. They would all seem to run together. I had to really stare at the keyboard to make out anything, and I'd get confused. I could answer the phone alright, but a major part of being a receptionist is being able to transfer calls without a long wait time. I know it sounds ludicrous, but I actually adapted by transferring all of the calls to a different department and they would transfer them to their proper destinations! Since they were doing my job, they weren't efficient in doing their tasks. It was one big mess, and I was always afraid it would blow up in my face one day and cause me to lose my volunteer position. I needed that position to help me fulfill a sense of purpose in helping others. Without it, I felt I would be worthless.

I wasn't proficient at my job until after I got my prism glasses. Now when I get calls and people are referencing a specific extension number, I can clearly see it, and there's no need for a panic attack as I no longer have to strain to see the numbers. Without the prism glasses, I was really concerned that I was going to need to give up my volunteer position because I couldn't fulfill the simple obligations that were involved. Now because of the glasses, I have the self-confidence, the motivation and the ability to continue doing what I love while contributing to my community by helping others.

I can enjoy sewing now, too. I can thread the needle when I sew and I couldn't do that before. I've been able to eliminate using the needle-threader. I'm now tickled pink that I can thread the needle myself. I can see the eye of the needle, and the colors of the threads I'm using. I'm much happier now making beautiful quilts. I excitedly showed another participant how I can thread the needle and he said to me: "That's no big deal—I can thread the needle too," and I replied: *"Yeah, but* you *weren't blind before!"*

J. Smith: I've referred several patients to Vision Specialists and if they aren't able to help them, they're honest about that fact. In some cases the eye misalignment may be so significant that what may be needed is a type of surgical correction.

I am one of Vision Specialists of Michigan strongest advocates now! I even took the initiative and gave a presentation at a health conference last year in an effort to disseminate this information to providers in various health care fields.

Bryan   I wish more people would have the opportunity to go to Vision Specialists of Michigan and get the kind of help they need. There simply are not enough people that are aware of this condition, making it that much more difficult when looking for answers. I want people to know that I was just like that. I had received a pair of glasses that just didn't work for me and I simply stopped wearing them. But I kept talking about the need to get glasses that would help me, and finally someone listened. That person cared and that person referred me to Vision Specialists and I was glad to have the opportunity to go. I wear my glasses everyday now. From the time I get up in the morning until it's time to retire for bed. You become negative when you can't see or perform basic, simple functions. These are more than just 'glasses' for me. People need to rethink their idea of glasses and discover what prism glasses can do for them.

I Am No Longer 'Just Surviving' - I Am Thriving

by Glen Hieber

While riding my 10 speed bike in 2003, I was hit by a vehicle whose driver attempted to make it through a traffic light. It was approximately 7:30 in the morning and as a result, my bike was pushed into the busy intersection causing me to be hit twice by a pick-up truck! As one can imagine, I sustained multiple injuries. In addition to the traumatic brain injury (TBI) and internal injuries, I had to have a cast on one of my legs. While I was able to receive the much-needed emergent medical care for my condition, my not having medical insurance complicated matters, and once my life-threatening problems were addressed and taken care of, I was released from the hospital.

Unfortunately for me, this was a period of my life when I was staying at a rotating shelter. Not having a permanent address and moving from shelter to shelter complicated my being able to maintain a regular treatment schedule (which was needed at the time). During the beginning stages of my recuperation, I didn't have anyone to assist me in navigating the various medical agencies required to get the care that was necessary.

While recuperating from the accident, I began to notice some persistent symptoms such as constant headaches, blurred and double vision, dizziness, and a feeling that my balance was not right.

While walking in the lobby of a facility one day, I got really disoriented and dizzy and felt myself falling forward. It all happened so quickly that I didn't have time to use my arms to protect myself or cushion the fall. My head slammed into the marble floor, causing damage to my gums and knocking out two of my teeth. Part of my rehab allowed me to get a pair of glasses, but I did not notice any significant improvement in my vision. I was still experiencing blurred and doubled vision along with migraines, dizziness and vertigo. I thought I'd just have to give my eyes and myself some time to adjust to everything, but even after a month I hadn't noticed any improvement. I was nervous about falling all the time, and in fact, had another hard fall a few months later. By now I'd had appointments with optometrists, ophthalmologists, neurologists, speech therapists - you name it, I saw them. It was hard for me to communicate what was going on and I was becoming frustrated with trying to explain to the medical professionals exactly how I was feeling. It was all too overwhelming for me to deal with, and at one point, one of the professionals working with me determined that I needed a case manager to assist me in making sure I was receiving all of the help that I needed.

I began using what is referred to as 'compensatory strategies,' which is a good way of saying I was developing ways to compensate for my new limitations. With my going from specialist to specialist and not being given any answers for what was going on with me, I felt as if I was simply floating in a sea of mass confusion. I started to lose hope that anything would change, but knew that I couldn't give up trying.

Finally, when seeing my Physical Rehab doctor, I was told that my symptoms might stem from a condition called Vertical Heterophoria (VH). It was explained that with VH the eyes were not aligned properly, and that the condition could cause many of the symptoms that I'd been experiencing lately. It was also explained to me that many TBI patients suffer from this condition, as the trauma seems to cause the eyes to become misaligned. My bike accident resulted in the initial TBI, and my two bad falls afterwards exacerbated it.

I'd thought that all of my problems began with my accident, but the more I learned about Vertical Heterophoria, the more some things in my past which I hadn't understood before became crystal clear to me. As I was growing up, I used to say I had 'crooked eyes.' It wasn't something I could do anything about, but it was difficult for me to focus squarely on what or who I was looking at, as my eyes were constantly trying to align themselves to bring clarity to my vision. Unfortunately people would say things like: "You have shifty eyes, you can't be trusted," or "You just seem like a shady, shifty person." In our society, strong, confident eye-to-eye contact is important when conversing with someone, but with my condition, eye-to-eye contact was difficult and I avoided it whenever I could.

By the time I was referred to Vision Specialists of Michigan, a few years had passed since my accident. After having been shuffled through the medical care system, from seeing one doctor after another and not truly feeling as if any of them understood my symptoms or why I was having them, I had mixed feelings about yet another referral. On the one hand I was reluctant to start my story all over again, but on the other hand I wondered: What if this appointment turns out to be different than all of the others? With all of the other avenues I had taken so far not leading to improvement, what did I have to lose?

My first appointment with Vision Specialists of Michigan was unlike any of my previous experiences with other doctors. Just reading the questions in the questionnaire brought out emotions of heartfelt kinship for me, and I almost wanted to cry. The questionnaire totally rang a bell for me, and covered a lot of the symptoms I'd been experiencing but wasn't able to put into words. There were so many symptoms on the questionnaire that described exactly how I'd been feeling, it was as if the questionnaire had been developed personally for me. It was very powerful for me to see that, and I realized that Vision Specialists of Michigan was exactly where I needed to be! I had the distinct feeling that now I would get answers to many of the issues that had been plaguing me, and that things were finally coming together for me.

Dr. Debby asked me lots of questions but more importantly, she took the time to listen to my answers. Because of that, she was able to ask even more specific questions related to my own personal history and obtain a better understanding of what I had been trying to convey to all the other healthcare professionals I'd met with over the years. Dr. Debby explained to me in clear, concise language what Vertical Heterophoria is and how prism glasses had the possibility of correcting many of the symptoms I had been living with.

Vision Specialists of Michigan was definitely central in my road to recovery. They were able to make my prism glasses so precise that I can now look people in the eye when I am speaking with them, something I was not able to do before.

I used to like having walls around me so that I'd have something to reach for to keep me from falling down. The first thing I noticed when I was given the prism test glasses and asked to walk down the corridor in the office was that I no longer had to walk close to the wall for comfort, and therefore I was able to walk faster and with confidence! That was such an eye-opener for me. I had forgotten how freeing and relaxing it was to be able to walk comfortably!

Prior to getting my prism glasses, whether I was riding my bike or riding in a car, the landscape seemed to just be whizzing by me in one big scary blur, triggering feelings of vertigo. It was a frightening experience and I felt there wasn't much that could be done about it. As usual, I simply tried to cope with it. I also had what I refer to as 'rigidity' - I didn't want to move my eyes because there was a strange pain associated with them whenever I did, and because I would experience dizziness, nausea, and vertigo, too. I tried to keep them as rigid (or with as little movement) as I could.

Other symptoms I had prior to getting my prism glasses were: Neck pain, unsteadiness when walking, some sensitivity to light, and as a result of all of those symptoms, I also experienced anxiety. Just imagine trying to cope with a multitude of symptoms as you try to go through your daily routine. It was simply unbearable. I didn't like to go to malls, and although I liked music, I no longer wanted to attend concerts, which was highly unusual for me. The environment just seemed too noisy and too stimulating. I just felt it was overwhelming. After learning about VH and its' symptoms, I discovered that some of my 'compensatory strategies' (such as tilting my head to see or hear better) caused the excruciating neck and back pain I'd been having. My neck pain and headaches were greatly reduced as a result of my prism glasses, and my physical therapy sessions were reduced as well!

I felt very comfortable going through this process at Vision Specialists. The entire staff treats people right. It's like you're at a friendly family reunion, surrounded by people that listen to your concerns and are not just willing to help you, but *are able* to help you because they have the tools to do so.

As a photographer, my art stems from my vision, how I'm able to interpret what I see, and the ability to articulate that as an end result through the rendering of my photos and drawings. I honestly would not be able to do that at the level I'm doing it without my prism glasses.

I love nothing more than being able to go for a nature walk, look through my camera lens, and shoot beautiful pictures of the world that is unfolding all around us - the birds in flight, the river rushing by, icicles as they hang from the trees during the winter months. Vision Specialists of Michigan has helped me to be able to do all of that and more with my prism glasses.

I am no longer just surviving, I am thriving!

The Military Establishment Must Find Out About VH

by Michelle Dyarman

During my deployment to Iraq, I experienced 3 head injuries over a four month period (two roadside bombings (IED's) and a Humvee accident), which led to a mild stroke. After all of these brain injuries, I began to suffer from many symptoms including severe headaches, problems with my equilibrium and my depth perception. I experienced a significant decrease in my cognitive skills, and I couldn't read at all. Despite being evaluated and treated in the military medical system for three years, an effective treatment was never found, and these symptoms continued to plague me.

About that time, I was interviewed by Daniel Zwerdling from NPR (National Public Radio) for a show about the poor job the military was doing diagnosing TBI's (traumatic brain injuries). On the show, I discussed my head injuries and the problems I'd been experiencing with my equilibrium, which caused me to fall down a lot, sometimes resulting in further injuries. I could not walk without looking down at the floor and holding on to the wall. My entire life had been turned upside-down.

Shortly after my interview on NPR, I received a call from Dr. Debby. She left a brief message telling me that she listened to the radio program and thought she might be able to help me, and encouraged me to give her a call. However, I had no idea who she was, and I did not return the call. She called a few more times after that, but I was skeptical - what kind of a doctor would be reaching out to me? Finally, my dad convinced me to call her because at that point I had nothing to lose, and it would be best to at least hear what she proposed. I was still a bit reluctant, but I spoke with her by phone and she proceeded to ask me questions about all of my symptoms. She listened to me and really seemed to understand what I'd been going through. During the conversation she was even more convinced that she might be able to assist me. She said that for someone who had given so much to her country, the least she could do was cover the cost of the exam and the glasses – all I had to do was get to her clinic in Michigan. I felt better having spoken with her, but without knowing anything about VH (Vertical Heterophoria), I wasn't quite convinced she'd be able to help me. After thinking about it for awhile, I reasoned: *"It's only going to cost me air fare, and it's not like she's going to perform surgery on me – it would only be an eye exam and a pair of glasses. It's the least thing I could do for myself to go and check it all out."* So I made an appointment, booked a flight and went to Michigan. In retrospect, it was the best thing I could have ever done!

Once there, her evaluation revealed that I was a candidate for the prism glasses. Dr. Debby took the time to explain to me just exactly what VH is, and how misalignment of the eyes can cause so many symptoms. I remembered having told the military doctors several times that my right eye felt as if it was reading higher than my left eye, but they kept saying that was impossible. However, Dr. Debby's testing demonstrated that what I was feeling was exactly what was happening – *one eye actually was seeing higher than the other eye.*

When wearing the prism test lenses in the office that first day, I felt like a whole new person! *I felt significant relief of my symptoms within one hour.* Prior to that day I hadn't known a thing about prism lenses or the difference they could make, and I had no clue of how much of a difference they would make for me personally. However, since having my prism glasses, I no longer take medications for my migraines (as they are gone!), and I have been able to reduce the dose of some of my other medications. My equilibrium has improved markedly – I do not have to hold on to walls and stare at the floor while I'm walking, and I no longer fall down. I'm even able to read again. I had no idea a head injury could cause VH, and that VH could cause all of these problems.

I know this sounds strange for someone to say of their optometrist, but she truly gave me my life back! I call Dr. Debby 'My Angel.' Were it not for her, I'd still be suffering from the headaches, disequilibrium and reading difficulties - the symptoms all the other medical personnel kept insisting were not there. I'd been told by the other doctors that there was nothing wrong, and yet clearly there was. Unfortunately, this isn't an occurrence that has happened with just me, it's occurred with lots of other soldiers. They go for medical treatment, but the military medical community doesn't recognize when a person has VH, and instead tries to convince them that there is nothing wrong.

It would be a much better situation if the military medical community (and civilian medical community, too) knew about VH, and if the patient got treatment right away with prism glasses, instead of being prescribed various medications and treatments that just do not work.

One message I'd like to share with people who may be a bit skeptical about all of this: see how many of your symptoms are on the list on the home page of Dr Debby's website (www.VSofM.com). If you seem to be suffering from a lot of them – if the website seems to be describing you – then take the Vision Specialists of Michigan survey. They will call you to discuss the results, and let you know if you could benefit from a specialized eye exam to determine if you have VH.

I Looked Fine But Wasn't - No One Understood How Awful I Felt

by Dr. Susan Stoica   *Story 6*

As a highly trained and experienced engineer, I worked very long hours within my company. I was the type of person who really looked forward to solving problems. I had a lot of fun with my profession and I loved what I did. The more complex or challenging the issue, the more I looked forward to being able to assist in its resolution.

One morning I'd gone to work to demonstrate some information to another colleague. It was February, and there was a patch of black ice that I wasn't able to see on the pathway that I was walking on. I lost my footing and fell, going from a standing position to lying on my back with my head hitting the pavement. While the fall left me a bit sore, I got up, and noting that the black ice is what caused my fall, I went to a nearby store to get some salt to prevent others from also taking a fall. Although I was being cautious with spreading the salt on the walk-way, I unfortunately fell again. The second fall was just as damaging, as I hit my head again.

I immediately began to have horrible headaches. Shortly after that, I began to notice other symptoms as well. I couldn't lie down completely in bed, so I began to sleep in a sitting position. In addition, I was no longer able to read properly. The words would appear to move across the page and I was unable to comprehend what I'd just read. Since my job as an engineer was very demanding and required a high level of focus and concentration, I was no longer able to maintain my position. In a matter of months

I'd gone from being the major financial supporter for my family to feeling as if I were a burden. I was completely disengaged from everything and my life was just in shambles.

My whole body was in constant pain. I started searching for relief by going to doctors in various fields of the medical profession. I saw chiropractors, doctors of osteopathy, doctors specializing in allergies, and was subjected to numerous tests over the years. I was aware of some basic rules that I thought would be helpful, such as relaxation techniques to relax my muscles, and getting more sleep for my body, but my symptoms did not go away.

After a few years, I was in so much pain all over my body that I just prayed that something would help me. I'd become so disillusioned, that at one point I'd even considered ending it all. But then I would think about my son, and I knew I could not do that to him.

The worse part of the whole experience was that no one knew how I felt or understood how badly I was hurt, not even me. I was still thinking that I simply wasn't regaining capability, when in reality I no longer had the abilities that I'd had in the past. And because my injury wasn't something that you could physically see, my family, in trying to encourage me, would say: "Just get hold of yourself. Maybe you just need more sleep, or you're just tired." At first I thought they were right and I would try harder. But even with the extra effort, I was worsening. One day I almost fell asleep while driving, so I had to give up driving – another major loss.

Things were getting pretty bad for me. Unfortunately, many people don't know they might have problems as a result of a head injury - especially if the head injury was not a major one. Suddenly they're experiencing pain and forgetfulness and they think that it's something physical, so they begin to undergo a series of tests, and the tests show up as nothing wrong. And testing for brain injuries in itself is difficult to do. Unless you have bleeding or swelling or some type of hole that can be seen, it can easily go undetected. An estimated 80% of head injuries go undiagnosed. An MRI would only see major swelling or bleeding, or if there were holes or gaps where there shouldn't be. But it's possible to sustain a head injury that doesn't show up on tests and develop blurred vision, vertigo or a number of other symptoms.

For me, I had the headaches, couldn't read, became nauseous during car rides, and if I took a ride for thirty minutes or so I'd have to close my eyes for most of the time.

Finally one of my doctors, an osteopath who was working to realign my bones, referred me to Vision Specialists. He noted that with my symptoms, I could possibly benefit from their services. At this point I was barely seeing clearly and I was ready to try anything, and because I trusted the doctor that referred me to Vision Specialists, I was more relaxed about going to see them.

I can tell you this: I remember a marked difference after my initial visit, and that was very important to me. During the consultation, Dr. Dubin did a really good job at figuring out my visual prescription. He noted that when I looked at an object, one of my eyes would look ever so slightly upward and the other ever so slightly downward. This was due to the head injury. The optometrist at Vision Specialists spent several hours with me. Since my eyes were moving so much as he was testing me, it was very difficult at first to determine the diagnosis, but he was able to finally figure it out. That was wonderful for me, because I could finally function again.

Before getting the glasses, I was getting worse and worse. I was not able to watch TV. In the beginning I couldn't comprehend what I was reading, and eventually couldn't read at all. Every letter had a shadow around it, and they seemed to be jumping on the page. My eye muscles were continually trying to adjust to objects and finally it felt like my muscles just gave up. It was like I was in jail. I felt horrible.

Once I was fit with the prism glasses, there was an absolute difference for me! Now I take pleasure in being able to read without difficulty. I can watch TV, and I very rarely get headaches. I can even thread needles!

I am so happy that the doctor I was initially working with was familiar with Vision Specialists and what they do for people who are experiencing the symptoms that I had. Going there has changed my life. And for others, going to the website and completing the survey could change their lives as well.

After 11 Years, I Thought I'd Be Stuck With This Condition Forever!

by Julie P.   *Story 7*

Approximately eleven years ago I was in a car accident. Since I suffered no major injuries, I thought I was okay, but within a few months I started to get really sick. I began to feel as if I were too queasy to keep anything down and always had the sensation of wanting to throw up, and this feeling didn't go away. Coupled with the nausea was a feeling of motion sickness. It's hard to imagine feeling like that every moment of each day, but that was exactly how I felt. As if that weren't enough, I became unbalanced in my walking and seemed to get tripped up a lot. This made me reluctant to go places - especially places that I wasn't familiar with. I was just too nervous not knowing what would happen. I began avoiding places that were crowded because it was too difficult for me to focus on keeping my balance. I can even remember at one point during that time my mom saying to me that I walked like I was drunk! Still, in my mind I kept thinking all of this would go away at some point, and I'd be back to normal.

All of the doctors that I went to over the years attributed my symptoms to an inner ear issue. This is common when you're focusing on problems with balancing, but none of the physicians were able to find anything wrong. For the most part, they merely tried different treatments or techniques, but eventually advised me that there was nothing they could do for my particular case. Over time my condition worsened progressively, and yet I still had no idea what was causing it or even who to seek for help.

Although I was becoming more and more discouraged in seeking help for myself, there was a part of me that kept thinking there *has* to be a solution somewhere. I began reading about medical breakthroughs in treating the symptoms that I was experiencing, and when applicable, would seek help via those avenues.

After years of going to various specialists and still not having a solution to my problem, I began to reason with myself that perhaps I would simply be stuck with this condition forever. Many times when I spoke with doctors about my various issues, it just seemed as if no one was truly interested in helping me. One unsympathetic doctor even remarked that I should just be grateful that I did not have cancer! While I could certainly appreciate his having to deal with people with more severe conditions than mine, his flippant negation of my symptoms was hurtful. I thought: 'Of course I'm grateful that I do not have cancer, but I also want to have my life back to normal.'

One day my sister heard about a neurologist that she thought would be helpful for me. He'd been known to 'think outside of the box'. It was this particular neurologist that informed me about Dr. Debby. He explained to me that she was an optometrist that was having a great deal of success in treating people with dizziness. By this time, due to my symptoms, I didn't feel safe driving. I was unbalanced and was using my hands to feel my way along when walking. I had the constant feeling of being extremely nauseated, and I had excruciating neck pain. Also, it was difficult to read because of the strain to my head and eyes. I'd been going to a well-known clinic for several years that was renowned for treating patients with dizziness, but even that clinic was not able to help me in any way.

One would think with all that I was going through, I'd be happy to give Vision Specialists a try. Strangely enough though, I put off going right away, because for me, it felt like the last hope I had for resolution, and I was afraid that maybe they wouldn't be able to help me. It was nerve-wracking just thinking about it. I kept thinking: *'If I go there and it doesn't work, then I truly have nothing left, and I'd have to resign myself with the idea of having to deal with this condition for the rest of my life.'* Shortly after receiving the referral from my neurologist, I had extensive time away from work and welcomed it as a great opportunity to focus on my health. I eventually made the appointment with Vision Specialist of Michigan and allowed myself to think of the possibilities it could hold for me.

Once there, it was unlike any eye exam I'd ever had. I realized I'd acquired habits over the years that I'd never even paid much attention to. Like tilting my head to one side. I assured Dr. Debby that was something I did not do, but it was quite evident that I do! 'How could I not have known that I do that?' I wondered. I'd always thought that my neck and head were totally straight. Of course now I was able to understand why I had such excruciating neck pain all of the time - after tilting for so long, my muscles were just in a continuous tense state.

After trying on the prism test glasses for about 15 minutes in the waiting room, I noticed my neck pain had vanished. This was a pain that I'd had for the past 11 years! I remember simply saying to Dr. Debby: "My neck doesn't hurt." I was so elated that I couldn't wait to get my first pair of prism glasses.

It wasn't long after I began to wear my prism glasses that my other symptoms disappeared as well. I no longer had extreme nausea. I used to have to sit on the edge of my bed in the morning to wait for my nausea to pass. Then I'd shower and have to wait again; and dress and wait again. It was such a lengthy process just preparing for work. Some days I wasn't even sure if I'd be able to go to work. Today I don't even have to think about it. I'm able to simply get up and go! For 11 years I'd been on medication for the nausea and now not only do I no longer experience nausea, I no longer need the medication for it.

The ever-present motion sickness is no longer with me, either. I'm centered when walking and I don't feel the need to stare at the ground. I can turn my head without getting dizzy, and no longer appear drunk while walking alone. In fact while out recently with my mom, she instinctively reached out for my arm to steady me like she used to do, and she was surprised that I no longer needed her assistance. I guess you could say my getting the prism glasses has improved my mothers' life as well, as she no longer has to run errands for me or worry about me like she used to!

I'm now able to drive more confidently. My night driving has even improved. And I can enjoy the pleasure of reading again (a luxury I hadn't been able to do in years). Before getting my prism glasses, just moving my eyes across the page felt nauseating.

It sounds unbelievable I know, but I felt as if I'd experienced a 95% cure - overnight! And to think it was something as simple as getting prism glasses. Now I can't imagine not wearing my prism glasses. I tell everyone I know about the difference they have made for me. I can only wonder how many other people there are out there that are doing the same thing I was doing: Going to different doctors and specialists, experiencing multiple symptoms, and not being able to receive any kind of relief. You'd be surprised how I've told other doctors about how these glasses have helped me with all of my symptoms and they just don't seem to understand. The medical community just does not seem to know about Vertical Heterophoria, but they have to be aware of the work in this area, so that they can recommend it as a possible avenue for people to explore, especially when nothing else seems to be working for them.

For people who are experiencing headaches, neck pain, are feeling unbalanced when walking, or especially for those suffering from dizziness: There is still hope for getting some relief - what if all you really need are the right pair of prescription glasses? We're talking about glasses here. It's not as if you'd have to undergo any invasive medical procedures. There are no drugs involved. It's safe. You're just going for an eye exam, which is something many of us do anyway, but this exam is very thorough and done in a comfortable setting. You'll be able to sit with the prism test glasses on, and if you have Vertical Heterophoria you will totally notice a difference. It's such a simple solution.

As for me, I'm extremely grateful that I was recommended to a neurologist who cared enough to refer me to Vision Specialists. That neurologist not only took the time to *hear* what I was saying, he *understood what I was saying and acted!*

So Many Pairs of Glasses That Simply Didn't Work

by Joe Horvath   *Story 8*

All of my troubles began when I was involved in a car accident. In my case, I didn't wear glasses at all prior to the accident, so everything that occurred in relation to my vision was totally new to me. I suffered a TBI (Traumatic Brain Injury) and as a result I was in a coma for 2½ weeks. Once having made it past that hurdle, I awakened only to find I could no longer see clearly. Everything was fuzzy and seemed to be out of alignment and I had a problem with depth perception and headaches. I was sent to the rehabilitation unit of the hospital where I started occupational, speech and physical therapies. I remember having to close one eye and squint really hard just to read a few words at a time.

I continued my various therapy sessions after being released from the hospital. I was still experiencing headaches and my eyesight was very poor. The occupational, speech, and physical therapists all were making note of my progress, and working as a team it was soon evident that they each were flagging similar symptoms: squinting really hard when trying to see, tilting my head, being somewhat off-balanced when standing or walking, and having double vision at times. I was sent to an eye doctor and was fit with a pair of glasses with bifocal lenses, but they didn't provide any real improvement overall. A year later I was still trying to adjust to them, and I was persistent in telling my therapists that there was still something really wrong. Whenever I tried to read, everything was distorted. My vision just didn't seem to come into focus and I asked to be re-tested.

Although the prescription for my glasses was changed, my vision (as well as my other symptoms) seemed to be in even worse shape than before! It was hard for me to focus on objects either close-by or in the distance. I still found myself having to squint in order to see a bit more clearly.

Eventually my occupational therapist approached me to give me information about Vision Specialists of Michigan and the work that they do with a condition called Vertical Heterophoria. The therapist had recently attended a presentation that Dr. Debby had conducted at the rehabilitation clinic, and she excitedly explained to me 'it was like a light-bulb turning on in her mind.' She told me she immediately thought of me when Dr. Debby explained the symptoms of Vertical Heterophoria. She asked if I would be willing to make an appointment with Vision Specialists. As a result of her recommendation and the information which she'd shared with me, I agreed to do so, but honestly, I'd been to several visits with various optometrists and ophthalmologists, and I'd been fit with numerous pairs of glasses that simply didn't work (and in some cases, only made matters worse). Therefore I didn't raise my hopes or expectations too much for that first visit to Vision Specialists of Michigan.

My appointment with Dr. Debby Feinberg was unusual in that it was the most thorough eye exam I'd ever experienced. I was impressed at how she explained everything she did and why. She asked questions about other physical symptoms I had as well (like headaches and my feeling of being off-balanced), not just those related to my vision. She calmly advised me that I did not need bifocals but rather that I needed prism added to my prescription glasses. She knew that I (like most people) had never heard of prism, and she shared with me basic information about the research that had been done in that field. During the eye exam, she made me

81

aware of what she was doing, while explaining the different types of prisms she was using to develop my prescription lenses. I was able to wear the prototype prism glasses around the office to see how clearly my vision would be and to see how I felt in them overall. They felt great!

When I went back to pick up my prism glasses, I put them on and it was as if I was able to see clearly for the first time in my entire life. Even before my accident, before ever having to wear glasses, I had never seen with such clarity! It was a totally new experience for me. The prism glasses seemed to have fixed every issue that I'd had been experiencing with my vision. I did not have to squint to focus on objects, my depth perception was corrected for objects near and far, I no longer had problems with reading and my double-vision was also eliminated. To this day when I'm walking around or driving I just take the time to look around me, just to realize how well I can now see. Everything is crisp and clear, and I see the world in a different light for sure.

For me, I just happened to have an occupational therapist who happened to attend a presentation that Dr. Debby Feinberg conducted. It was just what I needed at that particular time, and truthfully, what I could've used two years before. I'd been in the midst of seeing different specialists, being prescribed different glasses and was not able to find success with any of them. I urge people not to wait any longer if it's possible that they, too, might have VH. Visit the Vision Specialists of Michigan website and take the simple survey to find out if you're a candidate for prism lenses. You'll be glad you did!

My Other Doctors Seem To Think I'm Crazy!

by D. H.   *Story 9*

My story begins two years ago, on March 14th. That is a day that I will certainly never forget. I'm a reading specialist at a school. On that particular day, I was working on a ladder putting some posters up in a classroom when I made a move that caused the ladder to slip out from under me, resulting in my falling from a height of just over 14 feet. The fall broke multiple bones on the left side of my face. I underwent surgery on my face and mouth to put the bones back into place and repair them. In addition, I ended up having a closed head injury, and thus began the journey of which I'm about to share with you.

For six months I went to occupational, physical and speech therapies. These included psychological evaluations as well, to ensure my overall health. I started experiencing a severe sensitivity to light of all kinds, as well as a low tolerance for loud noises. I began having a lot of trouble with my balance in relation to walking and would become dizzy and lightheaded. I had difficulty being able to watch TV, and would become fatigued easily. I was no longer able to drive (which was a necessity for me). At the end of six months and having completed my basic rehabilitation process, I went through driving rehabilitation so that I'd be able to drive again and thus return to work.

Even though I was still losing my balance and continued experiencing all of my symptoms, my doctors informed me they'd done all that they could. I was advised that most of my symptoms were attributed to anxiety, which caused the dizziness that resulted in my not being able to balance myself properly when walking. I kept trying to tell them I was not feeling anxious, I was just losing my balance, but they insisted it was due to being anxious.

Driving was now a challenge as I had to muster all of my energy to focus on just that one task. I could do it, but I began to wonder how safe I was in doing so, as everything seemed to really fly by me at a high speed. It felt the same when I tried to watch TV. Everything seemed sped up as if moving at some type of hyper-speed.

I began to relay this information to one of the specialists I'd been seeing on a regular basis. I went over all of my symptoms, when they occurred and what I had to do to compensate for them, but still I wasn't able to receive any help.

Another six months with no improvement whatsoever had gone by. One of my physical medicine and rehabilitation doctors had gone to a seminar that Dr. Debby Feinberg of Vision Specialists of Michigan had presented, and he came back to speak to me about it. He'd noticed that as she talked about Vertical Heterophoria, she mentioned many of the symptoms I'd been having, and he thought it would be a great idea for me to make an appointment with her. He explained he'd begun referring some of his patients to be evaluated for prism glasses and he asked what I thought about giving it a try. I'd never heard of prism glasses before, but I replied that I was game for anything at that point. I advised him my major goal was simply to get well and to enjoy a better quality of life. I'd returned back to work by this time, but I truly wanted to alleviate (if not eliminate) some of the symptoms that I was dealing with. Truthfully, if he had asked me to jump, I would have simply asked 'how high?' So I was definitely ready to give it a try.

I made my appointment with Dr. Debby, who performed the most thorough eye exam I've ever had. I explained to her that other doctors kept insisting that I was anxious even though I was adamant that I wasn't. I confided in her that I felt as if the other doctors seemed to think that I was just crazy or something. They simply were not hearing me. Dr. Debby looked me straight in my eyes and said: "You are not crazy. What you're experiencing is not from anxiety. It's a condition in relation to the misalignment of your eyes." That was such a freeing moment for me! She completed the exam and fitted me with a pair of the prism test glasses and instructed me to walk down the hall, turn around, and return to the exam room. I felt really tall and confident just with putting the glasses on. I walked down the hallway and as I turned, I realized I was not dizzy! I thought: "Oh my goodness," and right there, I just started bawling. A complete, triumphant wave of relief washed over me from the realization that I'd finally found a resolution, and it was all I could do to express my feeling of thanks.

As I sat in the waiting room with the prism test glasses on, I was compelled to just keep looking around the room. Everything was so clear and I couldn't believe how great I felt. The difference was so dramatic for me that I was given a special prism clip-on for me to use until my prescription ones could be ordered and received.

When I got into my car to drive back home, I was so overcome with the fact that I could now drive with clarity, that I sat and cried for a few moments more. I realized that I'd been driving with a major handicap, and I was just thrilled that now, after all of this time, I'd been given a solution. Things no longer appeared to be flying by me at top speed. Once home, I called my husband and one of my friends to explain how elated I was.

Early after receiving my prism glasses, my husband and I went for a short walk. Normally I'd have to concentrate and really focus all my energy on simply walking. With the prism glasses, I was freed from that burden and was able to just enjoy the walk itself. I know for people who do that on a daily basis it is no big deal. However, when you're given that simple joy back into your life, it's a major deal. It felt much smoother and comfortable to do so. I hadn't felt that way in a long time. I'm now able to enjoy long walks, and it feels great to be able to do so.

Since I knew nothing about Vertical Heterophoria, I am also grateful to the doctor that was open-minded enough to recommend me to Vision Specialists. I've since learned that many years ago, it was thought that adding small amounts of prisms to lenses simply didn't work. We now know that they do work well, particularly with the many different symptoms that people may be experiencing due to Vertical Heterophoria.

Still, I spoke with a neurologist later about how the prism glasses helped me, and he totally disregarded them as being a catalyst for the improvement that I was experiencing. I was steadfast and told him of how I'd had immediate, quantifiable improvements with them and that they were indeed the reason why my symptoms had been eliminated and were no longer an issue for me. I know that doctors can't know everything in the field of medicine, but the awareness of Vertical Heterophoria and how prism glasses are helping patients definitely needs to be known. By the same token, I'd spoken with a different neurologist who is renowned for advancements in the field of neurology, and when I mentioned prism glasses to him, he was well aware of the difference they make for patients, and he gave credit to the work that is going on with prism lenses. I mention this because both doctors are in the same field of medicine, yet one was insistent prism lenses are not a solution to these symptoms and the other was confident about the difference it makes and continues to make for patients overall. At this point, most doctors do not know about Vertical Heterophoria, yet it is really important to find doctors that do.

Since obtaining my prism glasses, my visual acuity has never been better in my life! I no longer experience the feeling of being unbalanced. I can drive normally without having to feel drained of all of my energy because of focusing at the task at hand, and it no longer poses a traumatic ordeal for me. Even my reading has improved dramatically!

Another good thing about Vision Specialists is that they're about quality and not quantity when it comes to spending time with patients. For instance, Dr. Debby called me after I had my glasses for awhile just to see how I was doing, to ask how I was progressing, and to find out if the glasses needed to be tweaked or if I had any questions or concerns. That's the kind of attention I can safely say I've never received from any doctor of any kind. The entire staff is very authentic and compassionate towards all of their patients. They really enhance the experience of the eye exam, and you get the feeling that you're their only patient.

I'm a huge proponent of prism glasses. I recommend them to students and their parents when I see children tilting their heads, or who appear to be experiencing problems with reading or seeing. Ultimately their parents would have to follow up on such a recommendation, but if we as educators in the school system can head problems off beforehand for students, it would change their lives and maybe even benefit society overall.

All Doctors Need To Be Able To Identify VH Patients

by Holly B.   *Story 10*

My problems with Vertical Heterophoria (VH) started as a result of getting hit on the top of my head while working as an inpatient Physical Therapist Assistant. Initially I didn't think that anything was wrong, but after a few weeks had passed it was obvious I was having symptoms. I'd get really dizzy, at times feeling as if things were spinning around inside of my head. At other times it felt as if the room was spinning. I went to my primary care physician who referred me to an Ear/Nose/Throat (ENT) physician. She tested me for Benign Paroxysmal Positional Vertigo (BPPV), and the test was positive. She then sent me to a specialist who treated BPPV.

The BPPV specialist treated me for over a year, making the 'room spinning' dizziness go away. However, I was still experiencing episodes of mild to intense 'spinning inside my head' dizziness which felt horrible. The last time I saw him he told me that perhaps it was 'just all in my mind,' and I was advised that given the time that had transpired since the injury, and after having implemented the various treatments, there was no reason for me to be experiencing any dizziness at all. I knew there was something wrong, but no one could tell me what it was or how to fix it.

About five months after my initial accident I wound up having to take time off from work. When I returned to work I still wasn't able to function properly. I tried developing coping mechanisms that would allow me to function with the dizziness, but each day it became increasingly more difficult to do. I'd have to sit on the floor while working with a patient because I'd become too dizzy to stand. At first I thought I could just shake it off, push through it, and everything would be fine. But the more I tried to ignore my symptoms the worse they became. I changed jobs to a less demanding outpatient setting. I was able to maintain this job for several months, but eventually I had to quit working that one as well.

My problems with the dizziness and the feelings of spinning inside of my head began to make me afraid to venture outside of my home. I became unable to drive, fearful that I might hurt someone. I needed something to constantly hold on to when I was standing or walking to keep me from falling. I simply could not get around.

Almost another year passed, my dizziness continually worsened, and although my physicians were convinced it was all in my mind, I was sure there was more to it than that. One day while in my kitchen trying to cook, I had three eggs in my hand which I was about to prepare. I experienced a bad bout of dizziness and before I knew it I was lying flat out on the floor with broken eggs all around me. I had no warning and no way to protect myself from falling.

As a Physical Therapist Assistant I understood vertigo and had worked with patients that had it, but never imagined it would be something that I would have to deal with personally. I started doing research on the symptoms I'd been experiencing to see if I could find the right specialist that could help me get better. Unfortunately I wasn't able to find anyone.

One day a friend from church who was aware of some of the symptoms I'd been having sent me an e-mail saying she had come across some interesting information, and advised me to take a look at it. She sent me the website information for Vision Specialists of

Michigan. She thought it would be a good idea for me to complete the on-line questionnaire. The minute I went to the website and started reading about the symptoms of Vertical Heterophoria I said to myself. *"That's me. It's as if they're talking specifically about me."*

Soon after completing the questionnaire, I received a call from the staff at Vision Specialists of Michigan advising me that my score was exceptionally high, and that I might have VH and could possibly be helped at Vision Specialists. I was excited about the prospect of going to this appointment. Being a health care provider myself, I know that people tend to get a bit jaded or skeptical when dealing with the health care system because you see so many things that are promoting better health, and many of them don't work at all. However, Vision Specialists' website covered in detail so much of what I'd been experiencing that I felt I might have finally found the right place to get help.

During my exam at Vision Specialists, when I was asked a series of questions about other possible symptoms I might have had in the past, I kept saying: "That's me, yes, that's what I've experienced." For instance, even as a child I would love to get on the swing set, but after only a few minutes, I'd get sick and have to get off and go and lie down. Also, I could never ride comfortably in the back seat of a car - I'd get motion sick. I always had to sit up front between my parents. Rides at the amusement park? Forget it - I was always the one standing at the end of the ride holding the packages.

For me, the relief of putting on a pair of the prism glasses was instantaneous. During the pre-exam time at Vision Specialists, I had to run my hand across the walls to help my balance as I guided myself from one room to the other. After trying the prism test glasses, I was able to stand without leaning or needing anything to guide me. It felt good! I turned around to see how I would feel, and I didn't feel dizzy. I immediately thought to myself: *"Okay, you can't take these glasses away - ever!"* I was just amazed at how great it felt.

Thank goodness my friend told me about Vision Specialists of Michigan. Having the prism glasses makes a huge difference. Before getting these special glasses, I'd try to go out to my backyard to garden, but I'd have to go back into the house because of my symptoms. I was literally home-bound. I'm now able to walk, drive, and read without experiencing problems; and I can work with ease at the computer. I'm not 100% back to where I was prior to my accident, but the prism glasses have allowed me to make some major improvements in my life. I've since been able to return to work and I'm now teaching in a Physical Therapist Assistant program. Being able to enjoy my gardening is a blessing to me. People around me were able to tell that something had changed for me (even without knowing I had gotten the prism glasses) by the way I walked and stood and interacted with them. They could see that something had affected a major change with me. It was just amazing!

We need to educate the medical world about Vertical Heterophoria. More optometrists and ophthalmologist need to be trained in this area. Other doctors and medical professionals need to be able to recognize the symptoms of VH so that they can direct these patients to an appropriately trained vision specialist.

People need to be able to get relief from these symptoms in a more timely fashion. It shouldn't have to take two years.

I'd Been Sick For So Long And 'Just Like That' I Was Better

by Suzanne S.   *Story 11*

I was involved in a car accident, after which I began experiencing nausea, cold sweats and an overall feeling of being sick. Thus began my journey of seeing specialists to try and figure this out. Six months after the accident I continued to struggle with nausea, cold sweats, and a constant feeling of motion sickness. Not the kind that comes and goes, but a non-stop feeling of motion sickness all day. I felt so miserable.

I was referred to Vision Specialist by a doctor who I'd been seeing for a different medical condition altogether. She was aware of the problems I'd been having, knew of the symptoms of Vertical Heterophoria, and knew that Vision Specialists was expert at caring for people with this vision problem. She was convinced that I could be helped by them and she stated, "I know just where to send you." By this time I'd seen many different doctors and had gone back and forth to the emergency room (where they'd do MRI's, scopes, and x-rays), but no one had been able to determine what was wrong with me. By the time my doctor recommended Vision Specialists, I was so tired of being motion sick, nauseated and sweaty that I was more than willing to give it a try. I didn't have any qualms about going to Vision Specialist because I had a lot of trust in the doctor who recommended them to me.

During that first exam, when Dr. Debby put the prism test glasses on me and instructed me to wear them for a short while in the waiting area, I felt like I looked like the Terminator! I wasn't sure how helpful they would be, but I decided to give it a fair shot.

After about 20 minutes, Dr. Debby called me back into the exam room and asked me how I felt. It took me a moment before I replied, "You know what? I no longer feel motion sick and nauseated!" And then I put my hand up to my forehead and realized I was no longer sweaty. I thought, *'Oh my God, I'd been sick for so long and 'just like that' those symptoms were gone!'* It was a moment of pure elation for me. I expected that maybe over time I'd get some relief from the prism glasses, but it never occurred to me that it could happen immediately.

The prism glasses have made a major, positive impact on me. I had other symptoms that were apparently due to the VH (since they also improved when I started wearing the prism glasses). I no longer tilted my head (which I used to do), which helped ease my neck and shoulder pain. I used to occasionally hit a curb while driving. Now I could drive straight with confidence, no longer hitting curbs.

Dr. Debby is one of the most thorough doctors I've ever seen. I know most people don't expect to spend the time that is needed for this type of an eye exam (2-3 hours for the initial exam) but the staff at Vision Specialist are very thorough, and they really have a knack for fixing the major problem (VH) that is causing so many of the other symptoms.

When I was sick, I was not in the mood to see another doctor. I was too sick to research this information on my own, and wouldn't have even had a clue of where to look for it. I'd reached the point where I simply did not care anymore. I thought the way I was feeling was just how it would be for me for the rest of my life. I am so grateful that my doctor knew about VH and its symptoms and was able to refer me to Vision Specialists. But I'm concerned that others won't be as fortunate as I to get the help that they so desperately need if their doctor doesn't know about VH, or if there isn't a local specialist who cares for VH patients.

Prior to getting my prism glasses from Vision Specialist, I had difficulty with reading. I would skip lines or they'd seem to be missing. That was a huge problem for me because a part of my job was to read publicly and accurately. My reading had deteriorated so much that I wasn't able to fill out forms correctly, or comfortably read materials that were handed to me. I started avoiding situations where reading was essential. The strangest thing about all of this was that I actually did not equate any of this with a vision problem! I would just think that I didn't feel like reading, or that I was just tired. Now that I can see clearly again with my prism glasses I don't mind doing any of those activities, and I'm able to complete them without any difficulty. I've noticed improvements in many other areas, but the most significant ones are with my driving, my reading and my balance. Now I'm no longer sick of being sick – now I'm well!

I Have A Quality Of Life That I Did Not Have Before

by Brandy C.   *Story 12*

From my youth, I had always experienced migraines. Terrible headaches that were hard for me to cope with. Then at age sixteen I was involved in a very bad car accident. In addition to the many life-threatening injuries I had,   I also suffered a severe traumatic brain injury (TBI). As a result, I was in a coma for more than three months.

During my rehabilitation care I noticed my headaches were now daily, and they were quite debilitating, lasting throughout most of the day. The headaches affected my vision, my ability to move around, my thought processes - so many 'normal' areas of my life, preventing me from enjoying even the simplest pleasures. I was just miserable.

One day, my brother happened to see a television interview with Dr. Debby of Vision Specialists of Michigan, who was speaking about Vertical Heterophoria, its' symptoms, and the prism glasses that were helpful to patients who had the same problems that I'd been dealing with on a daily basis. He called me right away and excitedly told me about the program. The very next day I was able to call Vision Specialists of Michigan to speak with the staff. During the phone interview I was advised that I might be a candidate for a pair of glasses with the prism lenses, and an appointment date was set for me to be examined by Dr. Debby. In the interim, my grandfather assisted me in completing the pre-visit on-line forms on the Vision Specialists of Michigan website.

My grandmother accompanied me to the eye appointment. After the examination I was fitted with a pair of the prism test glasses to wear in the office to see how I felt. My grandmother instantly noticed a significant difference in my gait. Before wearing the prism glasses, when I walked my stance was such that it caused a choppy, loud sound when taking steps. As I walked across the floor, you could usually just follow the sound of my movements without even being in the same room with me, and you could pretty much pin-point right where I'd be. I also had a potential for falling as well. Wearing the prism test glasses, however, changed that. Though I still wasn't walking in a way that could be described as 'normal,' it was certainly a marked improvement overall. In addition, the prism test glasses allowed me to see more clearly, and everything appeared to be more in alignment.

The prism glasses have made a wonderful change in my life. Of course I still suffer from my brain injury, and I do still experience headaches, but they are much less severe and are not nearly as frequent. To date, I get them perhaps three or four times a year.

I had always been a voracious reader. I used to do math problems just for fun! After my car accident but before getting my prism glasses, I had not been able to read, and reading had been my most favorite thing to do in the world.

The prism glasses from Vision Specialists not only made a real difference with my debilitating headaches, but with many of my other symptoms as well. Even my family members noticed. For instance, one day I'd gone out to the garage to look for an item. I was out there for a short while searching, when my mother (who had been used to knowing wherever I was in the house just by hearing me walk) noticed she hadn't heard anything for a short while and began to frantically look for me in the house. She was relieved to find me out in the garage, and that was when she'd noticed the dramatic change the prism glasses had made for me. My usual choppy, loud gait had been replaced with my simply walking in a way that no longer caused attention. I realized the glasses had helped not just with my vision and headaches, but had also proved to be helpful with my nausea and with my motor skills as well. I now have prism glasses for swimming, another activity which I love to do, and am now able to do so much more freely and comfortably.

Prior to my serious brain injury (even with my grandparents having worked in the medical field) no one in my family had ever heard of Vertical Heterophoria. We weren't sure what to expect and did not want to get our hopes up too high. I couldn't comprehend that these glasses could make such a change for me, in so many areas. Since getting my glasses I have read almost 135 books within the last year! I'm reading, I'm swimming with prism goggles, my headaches have been drastically reduced, I'm walking remarkably better and my motor skills have improved. In short, I'm playing catch-up with all that I've missed in my life over the years. With all of the problems I'd been suffering on a daily basis as a direct result of having endured a TBI, prior to the prism glasses I didn't feel I had a good 'quality of life'. I can now emphatically declare that the prism glasses *have changed the quality of my life, and it is so much better than it was before!*

To Get The Kind Of Help I Got From Dr. Debby Was Providence!

by Randy Blausey   *Story 13*

My story begins with my car accident in 2005 that instantly changed my world. It took such a deep toll on me that for a while I didn't realize its' full impact, or what was really wrong. It just seemed as if my whole world was "not right," and nothing seemed to make sense to me. I'd begun to experience dizziness, headaches, a feeling of being slightly off-balanced, and I'd begun to sleep a lot. Combined, I just seemed to be in a state of total confusion and I didn't know why.

In my search to find answers I was very fortunate to have had a very receptive case manager who was aware of Vision Specialists of Michigan and the work they do. This case manager presented me with the questionnaire that is found on the Vision Specialists' website, and arranged for me to have my first appointment with Dr. Debby. Since I wasn't aware of Vertical Heterophoria (VH), it was highly unlikely that I would have ever discovered Vision Specialists on my own.

Initially my first response was that this was just another doctor on a long list of doctors that I have to go to see. But my case manager was really excited, so I was hopeful that this appointment might turn out differently from all of the others.

When you've been badly injured and begin to have to meander through the different specialists in the medical field seeking relief (or at least some answers as to what ails you and how to make it better), you can quickly see how some health care providers aren't really helpful. Without realizing it, some specialists are "listening" to you talk without really "hearing" or understanding your symptoms. Others make you feel as if your concerns are either not legitimate or just unimportant altogether. After a while of that kind of treatment, you begin to feel frustrated and you just want to be left alone. For me, that was simply the honest truth of it. By the time I was referred to Dr. Debby, I just went. It was what I was told to do, and the referral was made, and I didn't protest it.

Dr. Debby gave me a short questionnaire which to my surprise covered many of the symptoms which I'd been experiencing. During the eye examination she asked how I felt, how my eyes felt and if I had any eye strain when reading the eye charts, or during other parts of the examination. It was clear she didn't want me to 'struggle' to see clearly while completing the examination, so that the prescription she developed for me would be effortless and comfortable to use.

I'd finally come across someone from within the healthcare field who not only listened to my concerns and what I'd been experiencing, but truly seemed to understand me! After my first visit with Dr. Debby, it was clear that she knew what she was doing and that she had special eye exam techniques that made a major difference for me. I received a pair of prism glasses that were perfect for my situation. It seemed as if my world had suddenly straightened up, which really pointed out just how topsy-turvy it had been.

A number of major changes occurred with the prism glasses. Reading was now tolerable, as the issues of having to concentrate so hard and losing my place were significantly reduced. It took a bit of time for my brain to readjust to my new sight. I'd been leaning to the left quite a bit without being aware I was doing so. The prism glasses allowed me to make it down a corridor by reducing the problems of leaning to the left or of experiencing dizziness. Even so, I continue to experience some problems with depth perception which causes balance issues for me.

It was difficult at first getting used to wearing the prism glasses all the time. But then I began to realize that some of my symptoms related to my vision were abating. I had to go back to Vision Specialists a few times during the first year in order to allow Dr. Debby to reexamine my eyes and to adjust / tweak the prescription of the lenses to get them just right.

Speaking with the staff at Vision Specialists or reading the information on their website allows people to become more aware of the symptoms they've been coping with for years, and that they thought were 'normal', and allows the people who are suffering to see that they have an opportunity to not just develop a coping mechanism or a work-around to their symptoms, but to get to the root of the symptoms and reduce or eliminate them.

Dr. Debby is one of the few people in my life that has been able to make a difference for me since I'd been hurt in the car accident. Sometimes when you have so much that's wrong with you all at once, you simply want to give up. To be able to find someone that has the knowledge to make a dramatic change in your life is just astounding. That was the gift that I'd been given in Dr. Debby. She really cared and took the time to explain to me clearly what was going on, and took an interest in me as a person. What she did worked for me and made a huge difference.

I still have some of the symptoms that I developed as a result of having had my initial accident, but today with the prism glasses, the severity and degree of those concerns have been dramatically decreased, resulting in major changes in my life. The prism glasses I currently have allow my vision to become amazingly clear. When

I put them on, it's like an explosion of color and clarity. Whatever Dr. Debby has discovered and refined, it truly works!

Unfortunately, too few people are aware that VH is a real condition that can be helped with prism glasses. It is important to know that there are other optometrists and ophthalmologist that work with prism lenses, but they do not work with them in the same way that they do at Vision Specialists. Therefore people may be prescribed prism lenses with little to no impact and sadly come to the conclusion that they simply do not work. It's not a negative on their doctor (as this information is just now becoming available), but unless the vision doctor understands and utilizes the techniques being used at Vision Specialists, their patients most likely will not be truly helped. It is not a quick-fix. You will need to spend time to have a thorough eye exam, and you may need to have your prescription tweaked a few times, but we're talking about the gift of vision that has the possibility of alleviating or eliminating debilitating symptoms that many people continue to suffer from needlessly on a daily basis.

I am eternally grateful for having been a patient of Vision Specialists of Michigan. You can call it a gift or whatever you want, but to get the kind of help I was able to get from Dr. Debby in my life, was to me - providence!

From Needing Help To Walk, To Walking A 5k Event!

by Katie Brigmon   *Story 14*

My troubles started as a result of a car accident. I was driving when suddenly the driver of a truck made an illegal left turn in front of me and collided with my vehicle. Initially I felt blessed as my only symptom seemed to be a headache, but then the other symptoms began to manifest. I developed double vision. My reading comprehension was severely affected and I had to read something eight or nine times in order to actually 'get it.' Words seemed to run together. I became very sensitive to lights, making it difficult to even watch TV. I was constantly experiencing neck, back and shoulder pain. I had developed dizziness and difficulty with my balance and coordination which eventually became so severe I was not able to walk without assistance. When using escalators I'd get so dizzy that I'd have to have someone with me - I would close my eyes just after stepping on, and when we would get near the top they'd tell me, and I would open my eyes to step off. I became dizzy just bending over to retrieve objects from the floor. The headaches became quite severe. They were there every day, and it felt like I had a band around my entire head that was constantly squeezing, causing excruciating pain and an intense pressure or pull on my face. At times my head was too sensitive for me to even touch.

I realized my life had changed drastically. Prior to the car accident I'd been employed as a medical billing professional and I worked for a great company, but now I was no longer able to work. It was very challenging to deal with these new limitations, physically as well as emotionally. Over the next 18 months, I went to many different specialists including PM&R (Physical Medicine and Rehab) doctors, Physical Therapists, optometrists, neurologists and chiropractors, as well as a cranial-sacral therapist, and I was placed on medications for head pain, neck and back pain and the dizziness, but nothing seemed to help much.

During one of my visits to my PM&R doctor, as I was describing my face, head, neck and shoulder pain, the "light went on" for her and she recognized the set of symptoms as possibly being due to Vertical Heterophoria (VH), and she suggested that I go see an eye doctor that specialized in VH. I wasn't too thrilled with having to see yet another doctor, and I was very skeptical considering all of the other specialists hadn't been able to help me so far. However, since I trusted the doctor that was recommending me, I had a sliver of hope (but not much) and made the appointment.

When I first walked into the waiting room of Vision Specialists and saw some people with the prism test glasses on, I wondered, 'What the heck is all of this about?' It reminded me of a scene from Harry Potter because they kind of looked like the Wizard Boy from the movie! My initial thoughts were: Am I going to have to wear these things for the rest of my life? I didn't know at that point that the prism test glasses were just used during the exam in the office. I must admit, I was quite skeptical. I did not believe for a minute that those crazy prism glasses could help me. With everything else I'd been through with so many other doctors and specialists, I simply didn't expect much.

I'm happy to report that I couldn't have been more wrong – everything changed for the better after I got my prism glasses! I was no longer having double vision and the words on the page no longer ran together. I could complete forms now without the anxiety that was usually associated with doing so. The constant pain that felt like a tight band around my head had been alleviated, and that squeezing sensation around my face was now gone. All of my dizziness and difficulty with balance and coordination markedly improved. I now felt lighter - it's such an amazing feeling! I really have improved so much, not just physically but emotionally as well. Even my neurologist has noticed these improvements.

I thank God for all of the work Dr. Debby has done with me to alleviate all of my symptoms because without her, I don't know where I would be. And to think at one point I thought I would never improve! I was so fortunate to have worked with a PM&R doctor who was aware of Vision Specialists and what they do.

As a final point, I want to share with you a great example of my improvements. Prior to getting my prism glasses, I used to need assistance just to walk. Unbelievable as it sounds, after getting the prism glasses I was able to complete my first 5k walk! To be able to go from needing assistance to walk, to independently completing a 5k walk is not something that can easily be put into words. I thank God for Dr. Debby and Vision Specialists of Michigan!

I'm Not Imagining Or Making Up These Symptoms, And I'm Not A Drug Seeker – It's VH

by Dan March   *Story 15*

My story starts while I was on active duty in Iraq. While on patrol, my Humvee was blown up by an IED, killing two of my buddies and leaving me with a significant brain injury and many symptoms. I had debilitating migraines five to six days a week, and severe headaches all the other times, which left me unable to function normally. I was dizzy and my balance was awful – I had to use a cane when I walked to keep from falling. I was frequently nauseous. I felt disoriented all the time, and this made me agitated. I had light sensitivity and pain in my eyes. I was constantly seeing stars. My vision was no longer crisp and clear, but hazy and blurry – it was like looking through a fog. I'd lose clarity when looking at colorful objects. Even though I had vision problems, it never occurred to me that my other symptoms had anything to do with my eyes.

As a veteran, I was able to go to the Veterans' Administration medical system for help. While going to my appointments and tests, I met a man by the name of Rick Briggs, a vet himself who is in charge of the Veteran's Affairs section of BIAMI (Brain Injury Association of Michigan). He works hand-in-hand with the Veterans' Administration to help people like me get better. One of the activities he arranged for me to attend was the 2010 BIAMI Annual Conference, which was held in Lansing, Michigan. This is the largest meeting in the country for brain injury patients and the medical professionals who care for them.

While attending that conference, I was asked to be a demonstration patient for a doctor who was speaking about unusual causes of headaches in TBI patients, and I agreed to help. He and I were seated in the front of the lecture hall. He asked me questions about my headaches, and performed a neurological examination on me. I was then asked questions from members of the audience, which was made up of various professionals in the brain injury medical community, as well as people from the general population who were attending the conference.

At the end of the session, Dr. Debby and her husband, Dr. Mark Rosner, introduced themselves to me and explained that given the symptoms I was having, I might have a little known visual condition called Vertical Heterophoria (VH). Dr. Debby told me that for all that I had sacrificed for our country, she wanted to help me. She told me that if I could get to her office in Bloomfield Hills, Michigan (about a 5 hour drive from where I live), she would provide her services for free. This was very generous, and while she didn't know this, given our financial situation it was the only way I could come.

Although I was willing to be open-minded about going to Vision Specialists of Michigan for help, I was honestly concerned that it was just going to be one more thing to try that wasn't going to give me relief. I'd had so many tests and procedures done over the years that hadn't helped me, and treatments that hadn't worked, that I simply did not want to get my hopes up too high. Furthermore, I'd been told by some of my doctors that they thought that the majority of my problems were "all in my head," while other doctors seemed to be under the impression that my main goal was to obtain high-potency pain medication (a "drug seeker"). By the time I'd met up with Dr. Debby, I was understandably discouraged, and I didn't have much faith that anyone in the medical community would be able to help me.

My first appointment was very impressive. The eye exam was much more detailed than any eye exam I'd ever had (and I'd had plenty in my lifetime). While we were talking, she made eye contact directly with me – she wasn't just filling out paperwork and half-listening. She was tuned in to what I was saying and how it was being said. When the time came to wear the prism test glasses in the office and walk down the corridor, without realizing it *I was walking without using my cane*. I had it in my hand but I didn't need to use it. And when I left the office that day, *I simply carried the cane out with me*. I also noted that wearing the prism test glasses had an immediate calming effect on me. Furthermore, objects weren't so blurry, I didn't feel dizzy and the splitting headache I'd had when I first arrived at the office *had disappeared*! It was such a major difference from just one office visit!

I am happy to report that I have had marked improvement in my symptoms because of the prism glasses. My headaches are nowhere near as severe as they used to be. To this day I do not need to use a cane, as my balance has remained improved. My visual clarity is much better. I am no longer as anxious and as agitated as I used to be. All from a simple (maybe not so simple) pair of glasses!

Another interesting twist to the story involves my eight year old daughter. She had been complaining about headaches, and when Dr. Debby overheard this, she asked her some questions, and the answers led her to believe that she also should be tested for VH. It turned out that she did need the prism glasses. Since getting her prism glasses, her headaches have been less severe, and she has more clarity with her vision, and her reading has markedly improved. We're so glad to have found out about this early in her life as it will make a major impact on her life.

As far as we are concerned, we wouldn't be where we are today were it not for Dr. Debby. The difference with getting the prism lenses for our family members has made a major impact with us all.

Part Two

Stories From Children And Teenagers

A Severe Head Tilt Corrected With Prism Glasses

by Sue Lee (for Timothy) *Story 16*

Imagine going from specialist to specialist for your child, and having them undergo rigorous medical procedures - from Botox injections, to wearing a neck brace, to enduring a halo around their head, and to even being advised that extensive surgery may need to be performed. Then imagine being recommended to an eye doctor who not only discovers why the prior techniques did not work, but prescribes a pair of prism glasses that alleviates their symptoms and provides a clarity to your child's vision that they had not experienced before.

My son Timothy began experiencing various symptoms in his early teens which caused him to begin tilting his head towards his left side. The head tilt worsened over time, and was most evident when he was talking with others or reading. We noticed he'd tilt his head when speaking or listening to people, and at first we simply thought it was because they were strangers and he was a bit withdrawn and shy. Then we noticed he began to tilt his head when walking as well. We went to a pediatrician who thought it was just a habit of his, but it got worse and worse. He constantly tried to look straight, but he wasn't able to concentrate or see clearly when he did. Continuously tilting his head resulted in his neck being strained, causing pain.

In an effort to determine what was wrong with Timothy, we took him to a major university medical center. The specialist there told us his symptoms were all due to muscle and nerve strain. We were sent to all kinds of specialists to address this, from eye doctors to neurologists. Timothy was given Botox shots in his neck which didn't improve matters any. He was placed in traction for long periods of time (up to 14 hours a day) in an effort to relieve the neck strain. But when it was taken away, the head tilting and neck pain returned. At one point, he was even wearing a halo around his head. He'd had MRI's and X-rays taken, and one of the specialists suggested surgery (cutting of one of the neck muscles) might be helpful for him. In the interim, he'd been in rehabilitation therapy but none of these techniques worked for him.

Timothy's symptoms persisted and he continued to tilt his head when he was writing, speaking to people, or walking. One of his doctors suggested that we begin monitoring his symptoms to pinpoint when they were most acute. I noticed the only time Timothy wasn't tilting his head was when he was asleep. His head would be straight (which now makes sense, because when his eyes are closed there is no need to realign images, and therefore was no need to tilt the head). When I reported this finding, the doctor recommended we go to Vision Specialists to have his eyes thoroughly checked and to see if he needed prism glasses.

This is where the amazing part of our story begins. Within a few minutes of examining Timothy and asking some key questions, Dr. Debby was able to see that Timothy needed prism glasses. She had him wear prism test glasses and asked him to walk down a corridor. For the first time in years Timothy was able to walk straight! We were so excited we couldn't believe it.

When we were first told about Vision Specialists and the type of work they do, my initial thoughts were that they might be able to help in solving this problem because the doctor that supplied the referral seemed to be excited about sending us.

For Timothy, the prism glasses led to big changes on the first day. He had not been able to walk straight before, and now he was able to do so without difficulty or having dizziness. The prism glasses also relieved him of the head-tilting posture which caused the neck strain and neck pain he'd been experiencing. He was so happy to have those two symptoms improved, as these had been major problems for him. He stated he'd felt like a weight had been lifted from him.

I was so amazed at the immediate difference that I kept staring at him while he walked, because even though I could see it, it still seemed unbelievable.

Looking back, it appears that Timothy may have been suffering many of these symptoms over the years, but he'd managed to struggle through them and make up in areas where he'd been lacking, which is why he'd started tilting his head to compensate for the struggle his eyes were experiencing with Vertical Heterophoria.

We are so happy that he was able to be diagnosed in his teens, and not go through his entire life struggling to compensate for multiple symptoms that we simply did not understand. An important part of Timothy's improvement can be summed up in this story by what happened with Timothy afterwards:

> Prior to getting his prism glasses, whenever we went out to dine at a restaurant, Timothy would always follow closely behind us. Always. We simply chalked it up to his being shy and introverted. We had no idea he wasn't able to clearly see his surroundings. He was unsure of himself and stayed close-by. After he got his glasses, we went out to dinner to celebrate. Once we got to the restaurant, before I could even sit down, Timothy was out of sight and getting

his own plate and looking at the buffet items! He'd never done that before, but now he was sure in his steps and was able to clearly see his surroundings. He's confident enough to try new things and take comfortable risks and he feels good about all of that. He is much more sure of himself. It's only been a few months and he's doing exceptionally better in school, he's able to volunteer for projects which he couldn't do before and he's much happier than we've seen him in years.

When asked what the overall impact of having prism glasses has been for him, Timothy stated: *"I'm so happy that the issue has been identified and fixed, because it has made a big difference for me. I'm doing great in school and can now socialize with friends. I feel better about life and can approach my future with a much brighter outlook."*

So Many Kids Are Medicated For Anxiety And Depression When All They May Need Is Prism Glasses

by Mairi Clow   *Story 17*

I was diagnosed with Vertical Heterophoria in January of 2012. My right eye sees slightly higher than my left eye and my brain cannot piece the two images together. This caused me to have double-vision, no depth perception and constant movement in everything I see. The thing is, though, I didn't know I had vision problems. This being all I had ever known, I thought that the way I was seeing was normal.

I initially found out about Vertical Heterophoria (VH) when my mom and I were helping to set up a dance competition. We mentioned to the mother of one of the girls I danced with that I had recently been diagnosed with dyslexia. She told us that her daughter was dyslexic as well, but in addition, she also had something called "Vertical Heterophoria." She told us about the symptoms her daughter had and how treating the VH had changed her daughter's life. I had every symptom she listed off. My mother, who was sure I had it, took down the name of the eye doctor that treated it and made an appointment for me.

I was extremely reluctant to go to Vision Specialists of Michigan, knowing that if I did have VH, the only way to fix it would be with glasses. I used to wear glasses in elementary school and it wasn't a very positive experience. I grew to despise the way I looked in glasses. I thought that never in a million years would I ever agree to wearing glasses again.

At the appointment, my mother and I listened to Dr. Debby as she discussed with us the symptoms of Vertical Heterophoria. Those symptoms were almost an exact description of me. It was becoming apparent that it was very likely I had VH. It was then time to move on to the evaluation. Like any other eye doctor appointment, she tweaked my prescription by showing me letters on a sign and asking me which one was clearer - one with a lower prescription or one with a higher prescription. Unlike a standard eye doctor appointment, she also worked with my vertical and horizontal eye alignment. After she had tweaked the prescription to perfection, it was time to put on the prism test glasses. The difference was unbelievable! My eyes were tearing up in the hallway she had me walk down. I had never seen things so... still. Nothing could prepare me for the view that was about to come. I was taken out to the lobby of the doctor's office building, a room with windows where the beautiful landscaping in front of the building could be seen. When I was there, I broke down in tears, and if not for the doctor's arms that caught me, I would have fallen to the ground. I was about to faint out of shock, unable to absorb the world - still, dormant, and with depth perception for the first time in my life! I had never been so glad to be told I needed glasses!

The prism glasses have affected just about every aspect of my life. When I put the prism glasses on, not only did I see better, but I was talking louder (without the prism glasses, my ears falsely perceive my voice as being too loud); I was able to walk in a straight line and in crowds (without the prism glasses, I am unable to judge distances correctly); I no longer had a headache, stomachache, or pain in my legs (I didn't even know I was in pain before the prism glasses because I had been living with it all my life - I thought how I was feeling was what feeling "good" felt like); and the most amazing part of all, I was able to read, ACTUALLY READ!

For the first four days that I wore the prism glasses, I was too afraid to pick up a book because I didn't want to deal with either the shock of being able to read better or the disappointment of my reading comprehension and speed being the same as before. When I eventually did pick up the *Scarlet Letter* (because I had to read it for homework) I once again began to cry! It turned out I didn't have terrible reading skills - I just needed prism glasses! It was so overwhelming, I had to put the book down and just cry for a few minutes. When I opened it back up, I was reading like there was no tomorrow, and without even realizing it, I almost read to the end of the book!

I immediately asked my mom to take me to the library. I spent forever in the used books-for-sale room in back of the library just reading the backs of the books! My brother came back looking for me and found me lying on the ground with books all around me. He asked what was wrong. I laughed a little, and while trying to hold tears back told him I was fine - I was just reading. "The backs of the books?" he inquired with a puzzled tone in his voice. "Yes!" I exclaimed, "have you read them before!?!"

Since having the prism glasses, I have been reading MUCH more than I used to. I work hard to get my homework done just so I can read each night. I still have dyslexia. I know it is still harder for me to read than it is for most others. I know I may never be as fast a reader as other people. But this is still more than I could have ever asked for. I've been able to delete every audio-book off my iPod - something I thought I would need to rely on throughout this school year, next year, college, and the rest of my life. Reading was such a tedious and daunting task before the prism glasses, and now it is not. I don't know how someone can complain about assigned reading for school when reading is so enjoyable.

When I dance I wear prism contact lenses. They don't have my full prescription or the reading part that my prism glasses have. On one occasion I forgot to put my prism glasses back on afterward. I picked up a book to read and I couldn't make out what it said. My heart stopped. I started having a panic attack. For a while after getting the prism glasses, I was so afraid it was going to be like "Flowers for Algernon"- after being "cured" of my reading struggles, it would eventually all go back to the way it was before the prism glasses. I began crying, thinking it was over - the prism glasses had stopped working. After a minute or two, I realized I didn't have my prism glasses on. I took a deep breath and reached into my purse for them. I put them on, and instantly I was able to read again. I was okay - I could still read. The words I had been trying to make out were "they were."

Another HUGE difference the prism glasses have made is in my driving. I truly have no idea how I ever passed driver's training. Driving without my prism glasses is like playing the *Mario Kart* video game. My first driving lesson in driver's training was a disaster. I kept starting and stopping. People honked their horns at me. I was flipped off. I even ran over someone's lawn a little, much to the surprise of the man who was mowing it! I came home and begged my mother to let me drop out of the driving class. After talking it over though, I made the decision to tough it out. I did improve, but I felt my driving skills really lagged behind the other students in the class. I was one of the last ones to finish with the six drives required to finish the class because I was so afraid of driving. Luckily I made up for my horrendous driving with the written portion of the class, which I excelled in. Once I had my learner's permit, I used to get in fights with my mom while driving with her over almost sideswiping cars. I always thought I was a good distance from the other cars. Little did I know my mom was right - I was always right next to the other cars.

I've found it very hard to explain how I see without the prism glasses. Words are used to describe the relationships we have between ideas and what we observe from the world. However, not many other people have observed the world with vertical heterophoria and there are few words to describe it. What I have talked about isn't even the half of it. Describing what the world looks like without the prism glasses is just about as impossible as describing the color green to someone who has been blind their whole life - someone can tell them all they want about how it looks but without them ever seeing anything else like it, they will never be able to relate to it, and in the end, will never know what green looks like.

Then there is all the medication I have come off of. Plagued with anxiety and clinical depression almost my whole life, I always had to be medicated just to function. If I missed just one night of taking my anti-depressants, it felt like the end of the world the next day. It was practically a guarantee I would have panic attacks. Coming off of my medications was never an option. With the prism glasses though, the severity of my symptoms significantly declined. After a few months with the prism glasses, I made the decision to come off my medications. I won't lie; it was very hard to do. I had been on most of the medications since I was five years old. My body was reliant on the meds and freaked out when it was being deprived of the drugs it was used to getting every day. But with time, patience, and support from those around me, I have gotten off of most of the meds. I'm still weaning myself off of a few of them, but so far, the results have been unbelievably amazing. The difference is like night and day. I am more animated, more awake, more aware of what's going on around me, less "sedated," more social, and overall, much happier. *It seems the medications I was given by doctors to cure my illnesses were actually making my symptoms worse and causing more problems than they were solving.* My next step is to come off of the medications used to treat my IBS and acid reflux, which have also improved considerably since I got the prism glasses. *It's just sad how many kids like me are prescribed medications for anxiety and depression when really all they need is a pair of prism glasses.*

All I can really say to describe how Vertical Heterophoria has impacted me is this: it was like seeing without depth perception, everything was moving, and everything was double. There is so much more to it than that, but there is unfortunately, literally, no words I can find for it. It makes such a difference in my sight. EVERTHING looks different. When I first got the prism glasses, I found myself just staring down at my hand, perplexed by how different the lines on it looked. It makes such a difference in how I feel. I don't slouch as much and the head tilt I once had is gone. It makes such a difference that for a while, if I ever took off the prism glasses, I INSTANTLY felt nauseous (with time, though I have adjusted quite well to taking the prism glasses on and off).

The prism glasses have given me something I never thought I would have: the feeling I will succeed in college. It once seemed so daunting to think of all the reading I would have to do and I wondered how I would ever be able to handle it. I once had a psychologist ask me how I ever expected to major in English if I couldn't even read. I feel so blessed to have the ability to say yes, I can read now, and I know I'll be well off in college.

I'm so glad I found out about Vertical Heterophoria, and I hope that in the telling of my story others can identify that they, too, might have VH and get the help they need.

Mom: Why Did It Take 10 Years To Figure This Out?

by Carol Wall (for Julie)

As a parent, you strive to ensure optimum health for all of your children. This is quite challenging when it's discovered your infant is facing a multitude of problems. Ever since my daughter Julie could talk, she would say: *"My head hurts and I'm dizzy."* This from a child that wasn't even 3 years old yet! Along with the daily headaches and dizziness, she experienced motion sickness when riding in cars, as well as nausea and anxiety.

When she was about four, we took her to leading pediatric eye specialists in our area. At that time, we were told that Julie had one eye that was slightly higher than the other. We were advised that she was too young to have surgery to correct it, and that it was best to monitor things to see how her eye coordination developed. Meanwhile, she continued to complain of headaches and being dizzy on a daily basis.

Several tests were run, including MRI's and cat scans, and Julie underwent other medical procedures to determine the cause of her symptoms and what could be done to alleviate them. None of the tests showed why she was having such a difficult time.

Mentally, I'd tried to think of all the problems / conditions that could possibly be affecting her. We had her see a psychologist for her anxiety in the hope that techniques might be taught to her to help her reduce it. We changed her diet several times. We tried dairy-free and gluten free diets. She'd been seen by a neurologist that was also a migraine specialists who provided a medication for her headaches, but the prescription made her so dizzy that she wasn't able to function properly and wound up having to simply lie still for the bulk of the day.

I found out about Vision Specialists through my sister, who happened to find out about them through her neighbor Kimberly. Kimberly excitedly told my sister how Vision Specialists had been able to help her tremendously by prescribing prism glasses. My sister was aware that Kimberly had experienced many of the symptoms that my daughter Julie was dealing with. Kimberly was so passionate about the positive impact that her new pair of prism glasses had on her symptoms that after speaking with her, my sister called me immediately and told me that I needed to secure an appointment for Julie to see if she might be able to have similar success with prism glasses.

I called Vision Specialists and one of the staff there told me about the questionnaire on their website, and suggested I complete it and submit it for evaluation. I went through it with Julie and had her answer the questions accordingly. Shortly thereafter, we received a call from Dr. Debby advising us that Julie sounded like a prime candidate to be tested for Vertical Heterophoria.

By this time in our lives, we'd spent over 9 years searching for answers for some type of a cure for Julie. And it wasn't just surface searching. We spent years traveling to different cities and states, going from specialist to specialist, trying many different therapies. Over the years we endured financial tolls (we spent thousands of dollars) and endured emotional tolls in the form of having our hopes dashed when the consultants would say that there was nothing to be done; and when the therapies didn't work. Towards the end of our search, we underwent genetic testing in the hope that it might lead to answers as to why Julie was having these symptoms. However, her tests continued to be negative. She'd been poked and prodded for so many different procedures over the years and for the most part, she'd been a trooper through it all. Deciding to travel from Denver Colorado to Michigan for an appointment with Vision Specialists was not an issue for us. After all that we'd been through, if the trip had just the potential to decrease the pain level of Julie's daily headaches, we knew it would be well worth it.

When making the appointment with Vision Specialists, I was cautiously hopeful. I didn't want to get my hopes up too high. Once there though, and after spending time with Dr. Debby as she explained the entire process, it all started to make sense to me. I was beginning to understand that many of the symptoms that Julie had been dealing with over the span of her 10 years might be coming from a problem with her eye alignment.

Since her early youth, Julie had developed this head tilt. She'd cock her head to the right and look out of her left eye. Her teachers, family members and friends would always mention this to me. The first thing I noticed when Dr. Debby had Julie try the prism lenses on for the first time was that Julie's head straightened right up. I was watching this and I thought: "Oh my God, her neck and head are aligning correctly, and she's looking straight ahead!" Later, when Dr. Debby had Julie walk down the corridor while wearing the prism glasses, her whole gait had changed for the better. She was walking more confidently and straight and she seemed to be more sure of herself.

Soon, Dr. Debby had Julie step outside and asked her to read a few of the signs along the way. She asked how clear they were and how well Julie could see without having to strain to do so. She wanted to be sure Julie's prescription would work for her in all her visual situations. This was the most thorough and comprehensive eye exam Julie had ever had!

Prior to coming to Vision Specialists, we had been aware that Julie had double vision, and one summer she'd undergone vision therapy and I thought it had been cured. However, at one point during the exam, Dr. Debby had Julie remove her prism glasses and look at a sign that was close-by and had her describe to us what she saw. I was stunned when Julie reported: *"I see two of 'em!"* My heart sank, because up until that very moment, I had no idea of the depth of her vision problems, or that she was still experiencing double vision - I was surprised that this was still an ongoing issue for her.

After getting her prism glasses and being so thrilled with the immediate reduction of her symptoms, Julie looked at me and solemnly asked: *"Mom, why did it take 10 years to figure this out?"* I understood her query, and I sincerely replied: "Honey, I'm sorry it took so long, but I'm glad we found out now when you're only 10 years old. Imagine those people who went through what you've gone through for 30 or 40 years of their lives before finding out about Vision Specialists." Julie was then able to comprehend how lucky we were to be able to find someone that was able to put all of these symptoms together and come up with an effective treatment. She understood that this was what I'd been searching for and hoping to find for 10 years. I'd kept journals and logs and extensive notes on all of the different paths and avenues we'd taken to find answers. I always felt that someday, someone would be able to put all of these pieces together and make sense of it all. Who would've imagined Julies' answer would come in the form of a pair of prism glasses? Or that my sister, while just having a casual conversation with a neighbor who was excited about what Vision Specialists had been able to do for her, would call me and ask me to give them a try?

Of all of the questions in the questionnaire on the Vision Specialists website, the one that stood out for me personally was the one that asks if you feel overwhelmed when you go into a department store, or when you're in a crowd. In the past, Julie would always cling to me in those situations, and my friends would tell me I needed to do something about it. They'd remark that she was getting too old to continue doing that. But I knew it wasn't just Julie clinging on to me. I could tell it was much more than that, I just didn't know what - or why.

Julie loves wearing her prism glasses. In fact, during the first week she had them, she came to say good-night, and I noticed her prism glasses were wet. I asked what had happened and she grinned and said she'd forgotten to take them off in the shower! We all had a good laugh with that one. And once, we had to turn back to get her prism glasses on our way to school, because she realized she didn't have them. She enjoys the difference they have made in the quality of her life, and doesn't like to be without them.

Julie wanted me to share this message with you regarding the differences that she's noticed with her new prism glasses:

"I immediately noticed that things I looked at were bigger and clearer. I don't drift to one side when I walk now. After wearing the prism glasses for awhile, my headaches have decreased. They used to be as high as 5's and 6's on the pain scale and they were reduced to 3's and 4's and gradually they became 1's, 2's or 3's. That is a 50% difference in the pain I had before! I am now able to comfortably watch TV and go to movies, which wasn't easy for me to do before, because it would make me feel really nauseous (especially if the movie had a lot of action or fast-paced moves). I'm eating more now since I don't feel nauseous, and I don't get dizzy anymore. All of my symptoms have improved. The only other thing I'm looking forward to is if I could get rid of the headaches altogether. I'm happy they've decreased to the level I now have, but it would be great after 10 years to not have them at all."

As her mom, the improvements that I've noticed with Julie are many. Her head tilt is now gone. She has many more good days than bad, whereas before, it was the opposite. She's much more active. Her working memory and cognitive processing is getting better. She is no longer fatigued and tired after short bouts of doing an activity, as her stamina has increased. She's gained some appropriate weight since having the prism glasses because she no longer feels nauseous and is able to eat properly. It's as if her growth and development are now catching up to where she should be at this stage in her life. She's now doing all of the things she's always wanted to do, but was feeling too anxious or too overwhelmed to try. In fact, one of her young friends at school recently said she'd never seen Julie laugh so hard before and just relax and enjoy herself!

We've noticed that her personality is coming through more positively each day. She's more assertive and more sure of herself. It's been a real confidence booster for her. Her facial expressions have even changed! She's no longer so tight and tense, but more relaxed overall. Her teachers have noticed the marked changes with her and we're getting reports that she's more focused and more involved than she's ever been. She now interacts with other students and participates in on-going events.

At one point over the years, we'd decided that 'perhaps this was as good as it gets.' Julie had been exhausted from having endured surgeries, trying different remedies, seeing numerous specialists and with very little change in her symptoms. I thought, 'enough is enough. I need to just stop and allow her to be a kid for a change.' I shifted gears and resigned myself to learning how to cope with all that we had to deal with on a daily basis, and how best to teach Julie different ways to compensate as well, so that she'd be able to function independently once becoming an adult. I'd even given it a name. I called it 'Julie's Syndrome.' I thought if I couldn't know the cause of her symptoms, I could at least identify with them by giving them a name.

Upon first hearing about Vision Specialists, I felt it would be great to give it a try, because there were no needles to contend with, no blood to be drawn, no invasive procedures to prepare for, and no medications to prescribe. Vision Specialists has been great for our family! There couldn't have been a better answer. After our arduous 10 year search for answers and seeing the amazing improvements Julie has experienced, there are no words that can describe the happy ending to this journey. The prism glasses have given Julie a whole new life that she never had. Before Vision Specialists, I worried if Julie would ever be able to attend college and if so, how challenging that would be for her. I constantly wondered if she'd be able to be truly independent and live life on her own and to her fullest potential. Now I'm much more confident that she will be able to do all of that and more!

During a recent ice cream social to welcome a new family into the area, the major impact Vision Specialists has made for Julie was evident. Julie was so sociable. She didn't sit in my lap, she didn't cling to me, and she didn't become anxious or overwhelmed. She sat in her own chair. She was amicable. When she was asked a question, she looked directly at the person and spoke clearly and confidently. I'd never seen her exhibit that kind of behavior before. I thought to myself: *'This is simply not something we would've seen or experienced just 6 short months ago.'* She's still young enough that she hasn't missed out on the best years of her life, and she'll be able to catch up on many things.

What I would like to share with others is simply this: If you're experiencing the symptoms contained in the Vision Specialists' on-line questionnaire, don't discount the possibility that difficulty with your vision might be the source of your problems. The solution you've been searching for might be closer and simpler than you think!

Tilting My Head and Reading Problems Due To Eye Misalignment

by Rene B. (for Nicole)   *Story 19*

Imagine noticing your child experiencing problems with what appears to be their vision or hearing, which causes them to have difficulty or challenges in school, and the health care professionals you're seeing are not able to detect what is wrong. That is what was happening with my daughter Nicole.

When Nicole was in 1st grade, she began having problems in school with reading. In 2nd grade, she was diagnosed with dyslexia and as a result, wound up repeating the grade. In addition, she would always turn and tilt her head in a bizarre way when watching TV, listening to people speak, or trying to see the board at the front of the classroom. Her teachers noticed this, and thought it might be related to her not being able to hear well. So we took her to hearing specialists who conducted auditory tests, but they were not able to find anything wrong, and reported that her hearing was perfectly fine.

Nicole's symptoms did not go away, and being frustrated about it all, I happened to mention what I was going through to another mom at the school. We talked about the weird way that Nicole would tilt her head and how she seemed to have a problem focusing on objects when trying to see. This parent was also experiencing some difficult times with her own child at the school, so we would talk after school in the parking lot, and this led to us forming a friendship.

Nicole's symptoms worsened, and over the next two years we took her to different health care professionals and doctors such as hearing specialists, ENT (Ear/Nose/Throat) specialists and ophthalmologists, but no one was able to determine why she was having these symptoms.

Time passed, and now Nicole was entering 4th grade and things hadn't gotten any better with her symptoms. One day, the mom that I had bonded with a few years before excitedly told me that a friend of hers had a son who used to tilt his head a lot like Nicole was doing, and she told me that there was an eye doctor that was able to help them. She said she'd thought about everything I'd shared with her about Nicole's symptoms, and wanted to get this information to me immediately. She wasn't able to explain it all, but she did mention they used glasses with the prism in them to fix the symptoms. I was excited that this might be something helpful for my daughter.

I looked up Vision Specialists of Michigan phone number and called right away to make an appointment. I did not have the information for the website at that time, so I hadn't had the opportunity to see how all of Nicole's symptoms were connected, or the major changes that Vision Specialists' patients were experiencing.

At first, I didn't want to put too much hope in what Vision Specialists could do for Nicole. I just didn't want to set myself up for another disappointing defeat. I was a bit apprehensive, but not skeptical. I was just afraid that this would be something else that might not work. I was open to it though because I had a lot of faith in the mother that had shared the information with me, as I knew her to be a really genuine person, and since she was well aware of all of the different places we had gone to seek help for Nicole, I felt she wasn't exaggerating about how Vision Specialists might be able to help us.

With our first appointment, Dr. Debby did an eye exam with Nicole and I couldn't believe it - there actually was a reason for her tilting her head in such a weird way. I was so relieved that after almost 2 ½ years of searching for answers, someone was able to figure it all out. Things were explained to me in a way that I could understand, and it really opened my eyes and gave me a clear understanding as to what was happening and why.

During the exam, Dr. Debby was able to show me that when my daughter looked straight ahead, one of her eyes was positioned slightly higher than the other eye, causing her eyes to strain in order to not see double.

At first Nicole was too embarrassed to walk out into the office waiting room wearing the prism test glasses. She was just about to go into 4th grade, so she was really young and self-conscious. The staff at Vision Specialists was really understanding of her age and they allowed her to walk around inside the back areas of the office. Dr. Debby was really good at drawing Nicole out of her shell for the first few visits, and she knew just what questions to ask to get her to relax. It's just amazing how compassionate she is with her patients.

Before going to Vision Specialists and getting a pair of the prism glasses, there were things Nicole wanted to do but couldn't because of the different symptoms she was having. For instance, there was a talent show she really wanted to be in, and we encouraged her to do it, but she just kept saying she couldn't. She would have anxiety attacks and would become overwhelmed and did not feel comfortable speaking in front of groups.

Then in 4th grade, after she got the prism glasses, she really shocked me when she told me she was going to be an Emcee for the school's talent show. Sure enough, she got up on the stage in front of everyone and did a great job! I was so excited and happy for her. With the prism glasses, she felt more comfortable, self-confident and self-assured. She is a totally different person. She doesn't get as overwhelmed anymore, and she doesn't experience the anxiousness or nervousness that she used to experience, and she really feels that now she can finally do things she'd always wanted to do.

Before the prism glasses, getting Nicole to read was a constant struggle. I found myself nagging her to practice her reading and she hated it. She'd tilt or turn her head in weird ways to see more clearly, and she suffered from bouts of anxiety which caused her to not be confident. Mathematics was challenging for her, too. She would add the numbers sideways instead of up and down. She couldn't remember what direction the numbers should go in. These combined challenges were insurmountable for her.

After she began wearing the prism glasses, she experienced major improvements. She's more self-sufficient and she reads on her own without my having to ask her. She has discovered she enjoys reading and feels much more comfortable within herself. I can't imagine her having to go through middle school, high school or college without the prism glasses and the difference they've made for her. I don't know where we would be today without them. She's now doing things she has never been able to do before, like taking ice-skating lessons, and participating in school activities. She's more outgoing and feels capable of trying out new things. With the prism glasses, she doesn't have many of the limitations she used to have. She gets so much more enjoyment out of life now. My daughter still has the struggles with being dyslexic, but her eye misalignment just complicated things so much more.

A truly unseen gift was that Vision Specialists was able to assist not just Nicole with her problems, but was able to help me, one of my sisters, and a brother-in-law because we all discovered we had VH!

For me, I hadn't put two and two together on my own. I used to walk with a lean and I would joke that if I had to walk the center of a line for a drunken driving test I would fail after drinking just water! But I never thought it actually had anything to do with my eyes. I just thought that I was a little off-balanced. We have a normal tendency to adapt to what our weaknesses are and we don't think a lot about it.

As exciting as it was to see the major improvements with Nicole, it was equally as exciting to experience the improvements I was able to achieve personally. I no longer feel dizzy or nauseous when standing after having been seated for awhile. I used to dread driving in the center of a three-lane highway because I always felt off-kilter, but now I'm able to see the lines on the highway better and drive comfortably and not be nervous or anxious while doing so. I also used to have a fear of heights, and now I can look over the ledge without feeling as if I'm going to fall, and I don't have to grasp the hand rails tightly like I used to do when climbing staircases. At concerts or ball games I would always feel like I was going to fall off of the benches or chairs, even though I knew I wouldn't - I just *felt* as if I would. None of it made any sense to me. But finding out about the misalignment of my eyes and getting the prism glasses changed everything for me. Pictures on the wall look prettier. Colors are richer, everything is more crystal clear. I'm amazed at just how great I feel!

Looking back at it all, I feel I was blessed to have met the right people at the right time and place, because I otherwise would have never been given the information about Vision Specialists, and my family would not have been able to experience the major difference Vision Specialists was able to make in our lives!

School Vision Screenings Miss So Much

by R. H. (for R.)

The first sign I had that my son Rod might be experiencing problems with his vision was when he was in kindergarten. The children were paired off with what was called a 'reading buddy' - a fun, computer game reading program that beginning readers read along with. It had a booklet for the students to follow along. The computer would ask a question and the kids would verbally give an answer. Rod did quite well with this. One day while the two of us were reading the booklet at home, two pages were stuck together. He didn't realize it, and continued to read along as if the pages were in the correct order. He was saying the words that were on the pages that were stuck, rather than the pages we were actually turned to! It was then that I realized he'd memorized the book and wasn't really reading at all. I was floored!

We'd had him do the school vision tests each year for 3 years, and each time we'd been told that there was nothing wrong with his vision. I later investigated how the school system administers those exams, as well as what type of training and the length of training that is given to the staff that conducts the eye exams. Allow me to just simply inform parents not to rely on the school's testing results and to be proactive in getting a more thorough eye exam for your child (*see Editors' note). The earlier you can identify your child's vision problems, the sooner they can be addressed, hopefully preventing major issues.

I took Rod to an optometrist and when she put that first big 'E' chart up on the wall (which was in pretty close range for near-sighted vision) Rod stated that he couldn't tell what it was! At first

I thought he was kidding. The optometrist tried a few more tests with him and his answers didn't get any better. She then began to try different types of lenses with him in order to obtain his lens prescription. By the time she was done working with him she had tears in her eyes! She seemed to be half angry and half heart-broken. She spoke with me privately and advised me that to be legally blind one must test at 20/200. Then she told me that Rod tested at 20/400!

To compensate for his poor vision, Rod had become adept at learning in an auditory way. He'd memorized much of his schoolwork and reading tasks, giving us and his teachers the impression that he was where he should be in his development.

By the time Rod was in 3rd grade, he started having additional problems with his vision. During one of his eye exams, we were told that his eyes may be having a problem with convergence. It was noted that his left eye was overcompensating whenever he had to see objects up close. He was able to see in the distance well, but that was about it. His eye doctor referred us to an eye specialist in a different city, and Rod underwent approximately 6 months of vision therapy in an attempt to correct the overcompensation of his left eye.

After awhile it was clear that Rod wasn't making adequate progress with the vision therapy. It was discovered that his eyes were slightly misaligned. When reading he'd see the actual page, but he'd also see a transparency / shadow of the same page, which didn't allow him to see the letters clearly. At this point I began to wonder if he had ever been able to see letters clearly enough to associate them with their proper sound. It suddenly became clear to me why he was having such difficulty with reading. Anyone would under those circumstances. By this time Rod was about 8 years old. Rod's first pair of glasses were regular glasses, as we did not yet know about prism lenses. We were warned that he would need to go through an adjustment period (as his brain would now need to process images that he'd never seen before) and it may cause confusion and frustration for him. It was a journey of pure struggle, but after weathering through the adjustment period, the glasses became helpful for him and Rod finally got used to wearing them.

One summer Rod fell from his bike and hurt his wrist very badly. As he was being examined in the emergency room, he removed his glasses. The doctor that happened to be treating Rod noticed how he tilted his head and he asked my husband if Rod had always done that or if he'd just started doing that recently. When my husband called me to ask, I told him that Rod had tilted his head and squinted one of his eyes since he was 18 months old, but when I'd ask his doctors about it, they stated it may just be a nervous tick or something. They never associated it with a vision problem. The emergency room doctor mentioned the possibility of Rod having something called Vertical Heterophoria (VH) and told my husband of a clinic that specialized in treating that condition (Vision Specialists). I went to the computer to research VH, because I'd never heard of it before.

I found the questionnaire on the Vision Specialists website and I started going through the questions with Rod in mind. By the time I'd gotten halfway through it, I was just stunned! One of the questions addressed the issue of leaning or drifting to one side when walking and I was immediately reminded of how often I'd have to remind Rod not to run into me when we're walking together. I'd ask: "Why do you continue to bump into me?" He'd simply apologize, as he hadn't realized he was even doing it, and I simply chalked it up to his not paying attention to where he was walking. The questionnaire was very concise and the questions were so specific in such a variety of symptoms (of which Rod had many) that I was convinced this was something for us to seriously check out. Even when I was going through the questionnaire alone, I was reminded of various incidents that had occurred in Rod's life that I hadn't understood before, but the questions and the website information provided a clear explanation of what had been going on with him for years. For instance, when he was very young and we'd attend get-togethers or weddings where there'd be a gathering of many people with lots of chatter, noise or music, Rod would get so agitated that we'd have to leave. If we were having the event at our home, he'd get so overwhelmed that he'd slip into his bedroom by himself to be alone. For events where he was able to socialize with others on a one-on-one basis, he'd be fine, but among crowds or a group of people, it was just unbearable for him. After completing the survey I made an appointment with Vision Specialists.

During Rods' first eye exam at Vision Specialists, the optometrist had him walk down the hallway and I could clearly see him drifting to one side. I finally understood why he would constantly walk into me. We were asked if he gets motion sickness, and I recalled how he always had a problem if I turned a corner too sharply when driving. He always wanted to sit up front as he'd complain that sitting in the back seat made him sick. To realize so many of the symptoms that Rod had been having since he was an infant might be related to his vision was just astounding!

After getting his prism glasses you would've thought Rod was a totally different person! He actually showered in them! He swam in them. He didn't want to be without them for any reason. *He even asked us to take them off of him only after he'd fallen asleep!* That's how much better he'd felt wearing them.

Rod lost a lot of ground in regards to his reading level prior to getting the prism glasses, and we're currently working with him to improve his reading. I often think: Wouldn't it have been nice if the school had some type of system in place that would have identified Rod's reading problems? Instead of informing us that there were no vision concerns, we could have been made aware of his visual issues and made the necessary adjustments for him. He'd been tested at the ages of 3, 4 and 5, and each time we'd been told he'd passed his vision test. I wonder how many other parents (and more importantly, how many other children) are being given that same information when it is simply erroneous? (**see end note)

I was so upset about the entire issue that I attended a parent-teacher meeting and encouraged the staff to have a vision specialist trained in VH to do a presentation for the parents and staff to make them aware of what signs to look out for. Not surprisingly, there was a parent amongst the group that said her daughter had many of those symptoms.

When children are trying to learn to read, some are having major difficulties such as headaches, and taking much longer than their peers to cover the same material. The more problems they're facing when trying to learn to read, the less inclined they are to read. And who can blame them? Unfortunately reading is not an elective course. You have to learn that skill in order to live, to work, to drive, or to do anything. It's not a skill that students learn and don't use.

In Michigan, there's a service where dentists are transported in a big van and children are given free dental exams. Since in today's society you must be able to read in order to survive and to function in life, why can't they do something similar and provide eye exams that would determine if prism glasses are needed? Early identification of VH and other vision problems would allow for early intervention, which would prevent so many problems.

Having Rod hurt his wrist after falling from his bike wound up being a good thing for him in the grand scheme of things. I wonder where we'd be today had he not wound up in that emergency room on that particular day being seen by that particular doctor that happened to notice Rod's head tilt? Fortunately for Rod, the doctor was aware of Vision Specialists and the work they do with prism lenses, and recognized that Rod may be a candidate for prism glasses. This was a rare opportunity to change things around for our entire family. Strangely enough, the more I talk to people about the symptoms of Vertical Heterophoria, the more they recognize it in themselves, a family member or a friend**. Doesn't it make sense to see if you might be helped too? People need to understand that with VH, catching it early can prevent a whole lot of troubles later on, like neck and back pain and difficulty with reading and reading comprehension. You would be avoiding the cost of going from specialist to specialist seeking an answer, as well as the cost of prescription medications you would be told to take as you try to find out what's wrong.

People are unaware of the many health concerns that could be either prevented or alleviated by simply having a thorough eye exam by someone familiar with Vertical Heterophoria and its constellation of symptoms. *The right eye exam could have a major, positive impact in the quality of your life!*

{*Editor's note: a vision evaluation by a vision specialist who has expertise with children will identify vision problems that are not picked up on the screening exams performed in the schools or in the pediatrician's office. Please note that at this time there are no specific screening programs for VH.

**Approximately 5-10% of the population has VH – it is quite common!}

With Prism Glasses I Obtained Clarity Of Vision I Never Knew Existed

by Victoria Pace   *Story 21*

Looking back now, I realize that I'd exhibited several of the symptoms related to Vertical Heterophoria for quite some time. As far back as middle school I experienced neck and back pain and had been slightly dizzy sometimes. My lower back would knot up, causing severe pain, so much so that I'd started going to a masseuse while I was just in middle school. That would only work temporarily. The knots would come back frequently and my lower back would continue to hurt for no apparent reason. I remember feeling that I was too young to be experiencing all of this.

Back in 10th grade, I was walking down a hallway and for some reason I became really dizzy and I was unable to walk straight. I kept leaning and tilting closer and closer towards the wall. In fact, the hallway itself appeared to be tilted to one side. I'd always had a lean or a tilt, so at first this wasn't too unusual. Also back in 10th grade, I remember walking in the mall with my mom and several times she said: *"Victoria, you're walking into me again,"* and I didn't even realize that I was doing that. I also felt nauseated, and the dizziness started coming on more frequently.

Prior to having difficulty walking in the corridor at school, I'd been to my regular eye-doctor and had my lenses updated, so there was no reason for me to believe there was anything wrong with my eyes. Since there was no obvious reason why I was having these problems, my mom took me to a children's neurologist for tests to determine what was going on.

The tests were not conclusive and my symptoms persisted. We tried different doctors and underwent more tests, but they just couldn't figure out what was wrong with me. Around this time, a family friend had a son who was experiencing vision problems. He'd been prescribed a pair of prism glasses and his mom was so excited over the positive changes he experienced when wearing them (especially with his reading) that she suggested that it might be an avenue for me to check out. She had been aware that I had been getting dizzy frequently and was exhibiting symptoms similar to those that she'd noticed in her son. She felt sure that Vision Specialists would be able to help me tremendously, and she suggested I make an appointment with them.

While I was eager to do so, I felt a bit skeptical about going there because I'd experienced these symptoms since my early youth and wasn't sure if I could be helped. However, I was determined to be open-minded about the entire process because you never know what may be out there and available for you. Also, the family friend that had told us about Vision Specialists was really happy with the improvement her son had experienced. When she was explaining the symptoms he'd had, I noticed how they mimicked what I'd experienced for so long. I felt it was worth a try!

When meeting with Dr. Debby during the exam, she was not only able to accurately pinpoint my vision problems, but she was also able to describe my symptoms and detail exactly how they felt for me physically. I was rather surprised because it was like she really understood everything that I'd been going through all along.

Right there in the office, when I first tried on the prism test glasses, I noticed immediate differences. I was able to walk a straight line without getting dizzy or feeling disoriented. I'd always tilted my head in the past, but now I could hold my head and neck straight. I could swear it was as if everything was suddenly put into HD

(High Definition) for me for the first time! I never knew that objects had such definition and that things were actually meant to be seen clearly. This was truly vision like I had never experienced before! I was mesmerized with just looking around at things and being able to experience seeing in a whole new way. Colors appeared more alive and detailed. It really seemed that things appeared before me now as they should have appeared all along. I remember thinking: "Wow! So this is how we are supposed to be looking at things!"

There were other benefits for me including being able to improve my posture and sit up straight. This alleviated much of my neck and back pain, and as a result I have a lot fewer visits to the massage therapist. I still go to one, but the muscles aren't nearly as tense and tight or painful as they once were. My lightheadedness also went away, and hallways no longer seemed to be tilting.

Normally during class time, I'd have a hard time focusing and concentrating on my reading. My eyes used to twitch sporadically causing them to become tired, and I'd feel fatigued. With the prism glasses, this doesn't happen and I no longer experience those feelings. I'm able to concentrate better and be more attentive because my eyes are no longer straining and trying to compensate for my vision condition. As a result, I'm glad to say my reading skills have improved.

Before I had the prism glasses, I would have a hard time knowing when to stop when I was driving. I'd either stop too soon or stop too late. My depth perception was completely off, and I wasn't able to judge distances very well or measure accurately how far away something was. After getting the prism glasses my driving improved greatly, which boosted my overall confidence level (something that's especially important when you're a senior in high school)! For those times when it is bothersome to wear prism glasses (singing / performing / sports) I use a pair of prism contacts.

I can't give enough praise about the impact my prism glasses have had upon me. To say they've made a real difference is an understatement. I often wonder why it's not a requirement in a normal doctor's office to test people for VH, especially if people have had a concussion or any type of head injury that may cause them to have VH. There are so many things that could cause your eyes to be misaligned, from traumatic events to genetics. If it were a requirement or part of an overall preventative health care measure, it would have the potential to help so many people, and much earlier in their lives. I've mentioned to my friends (especially those that appear to have symptoms similar to what I had) how everything has improved for me with the prism glasses.

Part Three

Family Stories

For Me and My Family, The Prism Glasses Were More Than Amazing!

by K. S. & Family

During one of my usual busy days of running errands and setting time aside to shop for my children, I noticed that the day was gorgeous. The weather was great and the sun was shining down brightly. 'A little too brightly,' I thought, as I stopped by the doctor's office to pick up my new pair of prescription glasses along with a new pair of sunglasses. I alternated both pair of glasses throughout the day, making sure as I exited stores I'd quickly switch to the sunglasses to protect against its' rays.

Towards the end of my activity-filled day, I took the time to dine out in the early evening. Later that night I realized I felt terribly sick. My first thought was that perhaps I was experiencing a slight case of food poisoning after having eaten out.

The next morning I felt even worse. I opened my eyes and saw black and white speckles, the room seemed to be spinning and I felt dizzy. My symptoms didn't subside and I was quite ill for two days. I was too sick to get out of bed unless it was absolutely necessary. I felt fatigued and lethargic.

Thinking back, I remembered the only thing I'd done recently besides having dined out was picking up my new glasses and sunglasses. I wondered if perhaps the prescription was off by a little bit, or if my switching them so often while shopping that first day may have caused me to feel ill. When I spoke with others about that possibility, everyone said it must be something else and that there was no way that my glasses could be the cause of my new found symptoms.

Soon, my symptoms began to linger. My visual clarity wasn't there, I felt tired more often, I began to experience headaches and dizziness, I was constantly nauseous, and any type of bright light had an adverse effect on me. Sometimes I would get a tingling sensation along the nerves of my left arm. Eventually I had to stop driving. Even small noises affected me. I felt as if I were becoming a hermit, as I needed the lights in the room to be low, and was unable to tolerate even the simplest, low-level of noise. That can be a challenging obstacle when you're the mother of 4 children, three of whom are triplets!

Over the course of 6 months, I went to see various doctors and specialists to determine what was wrong, and what could be done about it. I received referrals to top-notch clinics and universities. In some cases this meant hospital stays while additional tests were conducted with the medical staff having me under observation. Unfortunately, these tests did not yield any answers for my particular situation.

I was left taking lots of different medications in an effort to see what might possibly help to alleviate some of my symptoms. I felt as if I were a guinea pig. Exasperated, I advised my physician that I'd completed much of the regimen and procedures asked of me, that I still did not feel any better, and that I really needed to find out exactly what was going on with my health - once and for all. At this point, I was given a referral to see Dr. Debby at Vision Specialists. Prior to my referral, I knew nothing about Vision Specialists, or the wonderful advancements they've made in the area of prism glasses for patients.

I felt so overwhelmed and at the end of my rope, that I actually called Vision Specialists from my hospital bed during one of my stays at a medical facility. I was determined not to leave there without first securing an appointment with Vision Specialists. I didn't know if they'd be able to help me or not, but I was desperate to give them the opportunity to do so. I was able to speak directly with Dr. Debby. I briefly explained all of my symptoms and that I'd been referred to her. I felt lucky that I was able to get an appointment rather quickly.

I came not knowing what to expect from the exam, and was pleasantly surprised to discover that with the prism test glasses I noticed immediate improvement! At the end of my appointment I felt as if the majority of my problems were solved. It was discovered that I had Vertical Heterophoria, a misalignment of the eyes which caused a multitude of problems for me. It felt so good to put on the prism test glasses and to be free of my symptoms! I simply couldn't understand how it could be possible for just a pair of glasses to have such an impact.

For me, it was beyond amazing. With the prism glasses I now had clarity with my vision. I stood taller and felt confident in my step. My first thought was: *"Oh my God, I don't want this feeling to go away!"* I felt great. My headaches were eliminated. I was no longer dizzy or nauseous and best of all, different types of lighting were no longer an issue for me. I was now able to walk in the mall with all kinds of lights from every direction and I was able to do so without any difficulty.

In hindsight, I truly wish I had known about Vision Specialist from the beginning. It would have saved me countless hours of going from specialist to specialist searching for answers. I could've avoided traveling to different medical facilities, undergoing various procedures (including a spinal tap and blood patches), and I certainly would have avoided the financial costs that were incurred as a result of all of that. Since my prism glasses eliminated my other symptoms, I no longer have to take the various medications I'd been prescribed - another huge savings in itself. I no longer have to wear my sunglasses in the house, noises aren't unbearable, and I'm able to drive. The prism glasses have literally given me my life back.

As a bonus, I took the opportunity to have my children examined at Vision Specialists. Their story began when I'd been informed by their school that two of my children had not been able to pass the vision test. Since I'd had such success through Vision Specialists, I felt it only made sense to take my children there for a complete, thorough eye exam. As it turns out, two of my children had motion-sickness whenever riding in the car, and one of my daughters (who loves to read) had difficulty reading while in the car. Other symptoms they had were eye strain, tilting their heads constantly and headaches from time to time. From of my own experience I was now aware that these were possible symptoms of Vertical Heterophoria.

The children wanted to take this opportunity to share with others the difference the prism glasses have made for them:

Victoria: I was having a lot of headaches with my old glasses. I'm a band student and sometimes my headaches would be so bad that I'd have to take my glasses off, which made it difficult to read my music. Also, I wasn't able to concentrate when reading in class. After getting my prism glasses, the first change I noticed was that my headaches went away. That made me happy! I was also able to see a lot better and my reading improved. I didn't have to take my glasses off in band class anymore, either. I was even able to do my homework with ease, as my eyes were no longer straining when doing so.

Austin: I wasn't able to see the chalkboard well, and words in books seemed really small, causing me to have to squint to see them. I had to read them more than once in order to understand what I'd just read. My prism glasses changed things for me because when reading, the words were clearer to me, and I could clearly see the words on the chalkboard without squinting or straining. I'm in 7th grade and at first I didn't really want to wear glasses, but now with the changes, I do feel more confident.

Vanessa: I was having problems seeing the letters on the board and wasn't able to read them clearly, as they looked rather blurry. I'm in 6th grade and I was excited about getting glasses because I was hoping I'd be able to see clearly and could feel more comfortable in all of my classes. Since the prism glasses, the blurriness is gone, and I'm able to even write on the board better than I was able to before.

Alexis: I noticed that when I would read I would skip lines, so I'd have to reread them. My vision was somewhat blurry and objects I looked at didn't seem quite clear to me. I'm in 7th grade and I like to read, but when trying to do so in the car, I would get headaches and motion sickness, so I wasn't able to read during long trips. After getting my prism glasses I was able to read without skipping lines. I was also able to read in the car without getting headaches and my motion sickness was gone. I'm able to engage in other activities in school now. My prism glasses make me feel a lot better!

Stories Of Those Who Had Symptoms As Children And As Adults

Either Something Is Terribly Wrong With Me, Or I'm Just Nuts!

by Carolyn Zucherrino

My first memory of experiencing unusual problems with my health was when I was about twelve years old. All of a sudden I began having dizzy spells. I remember my mom taking me to our family doctor who wasn't very sympathetic as he explained I was probably nervous about going through adolescence and that I was just stressed. I was given a prescription for pills to take whenever I felt dizzy, but when I took them, they simply did not work. Many times my mom would take me to the emergency room when my symptoms would worsen, but they weren't able to find anything.

My dizziness progressed over the years and by the time I was eighteen, I'd have to lie down when getting dizzy because I simply could not function. By this time, I figured something must really be wrong with me. One doctor I'd gone to thought I might be diabetic. I went through a huge series of tests to determine if that were so, but it turned out I was not. By this time my dizzy spells were severe enough that I'd have panic attacks worrying when and if I'd have one, where would I be if one occurred and asking myself how I would be able to handle it.

I vowed to act as normal as possible while trying to adapt to my condition. There were many incidents that I can remember as a result of it, but one incident really stands out. At nineteen, I'd been invited by some friends to visit Toronto, Canada to shop at this huge new mall. I was excited and eager to go. I had no idea that huge spaces would trigger my condition. In the middle of the mall, I began to have a severe panic attack. I didn't understand what was wrong. I'd experienced them before, but not like this one. It was overwhelming. I felt as if I would topple over at any minute. My friends wound up having to wheel me out of the mall, ending that day for us. My friends were really worried about me and I felt terribly embarrassed.

I began to attribute my dizzy spells and the feeling of falling to perhaps having low blood sugar and needing to change my diet. I thought to myself there wasn't much else I could do, except adapt to whatever was going on with me as best I could.

When I walked, everyone that I was with had to be on my right side. It was the same when I went to the movies. I was only comfortable if everyone was to the right of me, and if someone inadvertently wound up on my left side, I'd immediately correct it by repositioning myself. I was constantly being asked 'What is wrong with you?' At one point someone remarked that I was probably suffering from OCD (Obsessive Compulsive Disorder).

The years passed and I was able to be somewhat aware of when I would have another dizzy spell. However, I still had not yet found a physician that was able to help me. After I had my first daughter, I began to experience other symptoms. My neck and eyes began to hurt constantly. Along with my dizzy spells, I became overly concerned about being able to properly care for an infant. I was afraid I might fall on her while carrying her. This caused anxiety around the issue of motherhood for me.

At this point in my life I became completely fed up. My dizzy spells were no longer just three to four times a year, but I was now experiencing them weekly. They'd increased in frequency and severity and I had no way to combat them. My only rationalization was that I was truly sick physically or truly sick mentally. Did I have a brain tumor or something major league wrong with me? Was I completely crazy? I went to my family physician in tears to explain that I could no longer live like this. I stated: "I can't take it anymore. *Something* is wrong with me." After listening to me describe my symptoms, my family doctor told me she had a different doctor that may be able to help me with my dizziness and she gave me a referral to see Dr. Arthur Rosner, an ENT (Ear, Nose & Throat) specialist.

While meeting with Dr. Rosner I once again explained all of the symptoms I'd been experiencing, and how long I'd been dealing with those issues, and the various ways I'd sought treatment. He listened intently and when I finished, I was handed a questionnaire to fill out. As I began completing it, I thought: *'Oh my God, my whole life is being described on this form!* It was unbelievable, but there were so many of my symptoms laid out in black and white. The pain with my eyes, closing my right eye to focus, the neck pain, my being unbalanced when I walked causing me to run into other people, the dizziness, the tilting of the head, the vertigo, my anxiety and other symptoms. Over time, I'd attributed all of these things to my just being quirky or having weird ways and habits. There was a feeling of relief that washed over me that I cannot express. Dr. Rosner explained that he was pretty certain that I had a condition known as Vertical Heterophoria. He went on to explain that many of my problems may be related to my eyes and my vision. I remember thinking: *For all of the symptoms I'm suffering with, how could a 'cure' simply be glasses?* Were it not for the questionnaire I'd just completed, I would not have attributed anything to a solution as simple as that. But there was no denying all of the symptoms that were listed on the questionnaire that I'd been experiencing for over a decade. I felt I had to at least give it a try. He went on to tell me about Vision Specialists and the work they do with prism glasses that had helped many others with symptoms similar to mine, and I was recommended to see Dr. Paul Feinberg.

I'd worn glasses for driving or reading occasionally, so the idea of needing glasses wasn't foreign to me. I made the appointment hoping that since there was actually a name for my condition, someone would be able to help me. I couldn't help but think that this was my last hope.

After the very thorough eye exam, I was told that my Vertical Heterophoria condition was so severe that the staff was surprised I was even able to function at all! Without realizing it, I'd learned to adapt to my condition. While others at this level of severity had become depressed and weren't able to work or leave home, I'd plodded along day by day, developing ways to cope and continue with life as normally as I possibly could.

While wearing the prism test glasses in the office waiting room for only a short while, I was amazed at how much better I felt! I remember putting them on and actually walking without losing my balance. I stepped outside and noticed how beautiful the day actually was. I thought: *'This is what everyone else sees. This seriously changes my entire life!'* It was like seeing, really seeing, for the first time. Everything was crisp and in focus. The clarity was unbelievable. My eyes did not hurt. I couldn't wait to get my own glasses!

Many other positive changes occurred when I got my new prism glasses. I am no longer tilting my head and my neck pain has dissipated. I can now walk without losing my balance. My eyes no longer hurt. I can now walk into stores and actually finish shopping. Prior to the prism glasses I couldn't last in a Target store more than 10 or 15 minutes before having to leave. My dizziness and anxiety would simply get the best of me. Malls were out of the question. Another improvement for me is with driving. I can now drive at night since the glare from oncoming headlights is no longer a problem for me. In addition, the world of reading has completely changed. Whether looking at words on the pages of a book or looking at the computer screen, the words no longer bounce around so I no longer get dizzy or anxious as a result of doing either of those tasks. I realized now why working on the computer always caused anxiety for me. I dreaded doing it, and even checking my e-mails was a laborious task. The sad thing is, I'd always thought that it was just that way for everyone. It never occurred to me to ask others how they managed because I just thought that was how it was supposed to be!

I must say that at times I still get anxious, but that has to do with my own fears and personal thoughts. It's just hard for me to believe that it's possible I will no longer experience having dizzy spells, and I sometimes work myself into a frenzy thinking that they might come back. But I reason with myself that after so many years of having to deal with that issue, it may take a few years for me to get used to the idea that I'm actually healthy.

My mom is elated with the changes I've had since getting my prism glasses, because in actuality she'd suffered along with me over the years by taking me to emergency rooms, assisting me in searching for some type of cure, and helping me to function over the years. With my being a mother now, it deepens my understanding of what she was going through with me.

It's important for me to tell my story so that others like me can be helped – those who haven't a clue as to what's wrong with them and who just want to feel better. It's possible that you don't have a major illness and are not crazy or losing your mind. Who on earth would equate dizziness, headaches, neck pain and being unbalanced to just needing a pair of prism glasses?

When I speak with doctors about Vertical Heterophoria, most are not even aware of it, so it's no surprise that the average person doesn't know about it at all. I just look at my own case and am amazed at how I found out about it, with my family doctor recommending me to an ENT, who then recommended me to Vision Specialists. It is such a simple fix that it seemed almost too good to be true. This information should be on news shows that feature health topics and on shows like the *'Today Show'* in order to make as many people aware of it within as short a time frame as possible. The information needs to be prevalent enough so that Vertical Heterophoria is no longer 'new news' to people.

Until then, I strongly encourage others to visit the Vision Specialists website and fill out the questionnaire. No matter to what degree you're experiencing symptoms, see if you too, may be a candidate for prism glasses. Like me, it may seriously change your entire life!

Who Knew Eye Problems Could Cause These Drastic Symptoms?

by Karen Zakarian   *Story 24*

My story is quite unique, due to the degree of severity of the symptoms I was experiencing. One morning I woke up and before I even opened my eyes, I felt like I was 'spinning.' The only way to explain it clearly is: It was as if I was on one of those carousels that kids play on in the park, where one kid pushes it round and round while the other kids are on it. The faster it goes, the dizzier you get. Only I was feeling like that while still lying in my bed with my eyes closed!

I was so dizzy that I actually was not able to stand up. I had to go to the restroom on my hands and knees! In a mere 24 hour period, I'd gone from being able-bodied to not even being able to shower, because to shower you have to be able to stand. I was now bedridden and did not have a clue as to what had happened. The entire thing was just so bizarre to me.

Since the dizziness was believed to be caused by an inner ear issue, we went to a top ear institute in Michigan and worked with a specialist there. Unfortunately, they were not able to pinpoint what was causing my problem and were not able to bring me any relief.

Weeks were passing and my condition had not changed. I was not able to bathe, brush my teeth properly, or take care of myself. My condition was worsening (as I was beginning to have anxiety) and yet I was no closer to receiving any answers as to what was happening to me or why.

My fiancé had a friend who told him that her dad had experienced some of the same symptoms that I was going through, just not as severe. She explained that her father discovered that it was all due to a problem with his eyes. She told my fiancé about Vision Specialists and advised him that we should check it out. Of course we didn't think these drastic symptoms could in any way be related to my eyes, so we didn't look any further into that piece of information at that time.

After about a week with me not getting any better, my fiancé came to me and said he had a strong feeling that we should check out the information we'd been given about Dr. Debby and Vision Specialists. Together we reviewed the information on the Vision Specialists website and decided to give them a call.

My fiancé explained to Dr. Debby how severe my case was and we were able to secure an appointment in a relatively short period of time.

Through the questions that Dr. Debby asked me, we identified symptoms I'd had from my childhood that I'd never paid much attention to before now. For instance, in grade school I wasn't able to have school pictures taken because I was too sensitive to the bright lights. I wasn't able to go on some of the school trips like museums because of the lighting used in those buildings, and I wasn't able to even be outside for too long on the school grounds. I also recalled having motion sickness a lot when traveling as well.

I realized, too, that in college I would tilt my head to one side to try to accommodate my vision limitations. I was a dance minor in college, but I remembered never being able to do the turns correctly. I would try to focus on a point across the room in order to complete a specific turn and I simply couldn't do it and I never knew why. I would just get so dizzy and it would upset me terribly.

I reasoned that no one else was having trouble with the turns and I shouldn't be experiencing problems either. I began to wonder if there was simply something wrong with me. It affected my self-confidence. Again, I didn't think much of these things at the time, as I was merely doing what was necessary to continue on with my life.

As I got older and started to work, I would often experience a pain that felt like a pulling behind my right eye down the back of the right side of my neck and down to my scapula. I attributed all of this to my being on the computer for long hours at work. In my effort to resolve some of that stress, I had an ergonomic evaluation done at work. As you can see, I was desperately trying to not just adapt to my limitations, but to really discern what was going on, in an attempt to get things resolved. It would never have occurred to me that these issues were related to my eyes.

Initially, on that ill-fated morning when I awakened feeling as if I'd been spinning on a carousel, I rationalized to myself what must have occurred. That Friday, my office at work was getting painted and I'd become dizzy and had to leave early. I was thinking that it might be chemical toxicity, and knowing I was sensitive to that type of thing, I attributed my dizziness to the paint fumes. In addition, that evening I'd gone out with my fiancé to a Vietnamese restaurant. Afterwards, I could feel this deep, throbbing pain behind my right eye and down the right side of my neck, and I remember thinking that my overall symptoms were just a combination of the paint fumes and perhaps some MSG in some of the food that I had eaten.

I believe in holistic approaches to health care, so when I first started to experience my symptoms, we drove quite a distance to try a holistic approach to resolve them. I underwent a procedure that used low-level lasers but it wasn't helpful at all. As my

165

condition worsened, I went to a few other specialists, and while some of the remedies prescribed were temporarily helpful, they did not last.

So here we were at Vision Specialists for my initial appointment. I am convinced my case is perhaps one of the worse they have ever seen. By this time, I'd been bedridden for a total of five weeks. During that entire period, the only time I'd left my bed was to crawl to the restroom. I hadn't been able to shower prior to coming in and I was a total wreck.

Dr. Debby was understanding and gracious enough to do some of the testing with me lying flat on the floor because I was too dizzy to stand. Then for me, a miracle occurred right there in the office. After being fitted with the prism lenses, I was able to not only stand on my own, but walk in a straight line down the office corridor! When I came for my appointment, I wasn't sure how much she would be able to help my condition, and I was skeptical. However, the fact that I could now walk on my own again left me amazed! I was so thrilled that I began praising God right there in her office. My fiancé and I just couldn't believe this instantaneous difference - that in one visit I was able to stand and walk without assistance and not be dizzy or feel as if I were on a carousel! We were overjoyed!

My first pair of prism glasses allowed me to do many things, but I did need a few more appointments to get the prescription just right for me. Since getting my final pair of prism glasses, I've learned to drive again, and now it is without the anxiety and the dizziness.

It was coincidental that I was visiting Michigan at the time my symptoms began. I truly believe that most things happen for a reason. Had I been home in Chicago when all of these symptoms began to occur, there's a strong possibility that I would never have heard about Vision Specialists of Michigan, and could still be bed-ridden today. I'm not sure if there are any centers in Chicago that are even aware of Vertical Heterophoria [Editors note: as of now there are not]. As it were, I was bedridden here in Michigan for four weeks before we had even found out about Vision Specialists. During that entire time I only got out of bed to use the restroom and even then, it was on my hands and knees.

That's why it's important for me to share this story. Circumstances allowed me to be diagnosed and treated. But other people have been suffering for decades with no relief and no way to even hear about Vision Specialists and the important breakthroughs they've made in diagnosing and treating Vertical Heterophoria.

I now know why I suffered the symptoms I endured in grade school, high school and college. While it doesn't change that part of my life, it certainly has lifted the veil of uncertainty that surrounded me during that time. I've learned that with Vertical Heterophoria, one eye fights to align with the other eye and after so many years, your world can come crashing down around you without your having a clue what's wrong or how to fix it.

In my case, you can certainly say without prejudice that Vision Specialists brought my quality of life back to me - from being bedridden and crawling to the restroom on my hands and knees, to walking in a straight line and eventually being able to drive again!

I'm really looking forward to other optometrists and ophthalmologists getting thoroughly trained in the area of Vertical Heterophoria and being able to help their patients obtain greater levels of relief from the various symptoms they may be experiencing. I'd encourage others to visit the Vision Specialists website and simply take the survey, no matter what level or degree of VH symptoms that you are experiencing.

Wow! I Never Knew You Could Feel This Good Everyday!

by Jasmine Walton   *Story 25*

I remember having problems with my eyes as far back as elementary school. I had a difficult time seeing the chalkboard in class. I would complain to my mom that the boards were blurry and that I was having pain behind my eyes. My mom took me to an eye doctor who did a regular eye exam and explained to us that my eyes were fine, and prescribed eye drops. The eye doctor talked with my mom about her own history and as it turns out, my mom had migraines a lot and so did her mother.

As I got older, I was a bit apprehensive about taking the driver's test because I had concerns about seeing things in the distance clearly. But I managed to pass the test and continued on with my daily life. As the years passed by, I adapted to my shortcomings but I had that sinking feeling that there was something that wasn't quite right. I always thought my symptoms were related to my eyes, but I wasn't able to prove it.

While seeing a neurologist for other issues, I mentioned that I'd get headaches, blurry vision and experience dizziness while reading, and shared with him that working on the computer was even worse. I was eventually sent to an eye specialist, and was given a pair of reading glasses that didn't help with the eye strain or any of my other symptoms. After a couple of fruitless weeks I gave up on trying to use them.

During this time, I was no longer working, due not just to the issues I'd been experiencing with my eyes, but other health concerns as well. I had neck and back pain; I had no tolerance for certain kinds of lights or lighting; and many fragrances caused me to experience terrible headaches. I really needed someone to figure all of this out and help me get back to health, and back to work.

I tried to just be like everyone else and deal with my daily life, but it was challenging. One time, in an attempt to try to treat my symptoms, I accidentally over-medicated myself and wound up in the emergency room. Sometimes the headaches would be so bad I'd have to go to the ER for pain medicines. I'd begun to see different specialists for the various symptoms I was having, but they'd make me feel bad by stating that what I was experiencing was all in my head. Some of them didn't understand the degree of chemical sensitivity I had or the other issues I complained about.

For me socially, because I was always saying I couldn't be a part of things, friends had stopped calling to invite me out. It was very difficult for me to go out and interact with others because the various fragrances that people wore triggered my other symptoms and I just couldn't handle it. I'd gotten to the point where I was pretty isolated.

One day, my husband just happened to be communicating with someone on the computer who mentioned they'd experienced many of the same symptoms I was having. They told him about Vision Specialists of Michigan and how they were truly helped by them. They'd been really excited and gave high praise about the work this clinic was doing in the area of Vertical Heterophoria, and while recommending it to my husband, said it was something we should check out as well.

Since I wasn't working anymore, I began to feel like a burden on my family and started to become depressed. When I heard about Vision Specialists I was more than ready to check it out.

My husband talked with me about it and we went on-line to get more information about Vision Specialists and Vertical Heterophoria. Since they are located in Michigan and we live in California, we thought we'd first try to locate an eye doctor in our area that specialized in that field; however, we weren't able to find anyone locally. We decided I'd complete the survey listed on Vision Specialists' website and wait to hear from them directly.

I received a call from Dr. Debby shortly after completing the survey, and after speaking with her it appeared I was a candidate for the prism glasses she prescribes. We set an appointment for me to travel to Michigan for an eye exam, with the hope that a pair of these unique prism glasses might be able to help me.

The thought of getting on a plane in California and heading out to Michigan made me anxious. I was afraid I'd get a bad headache or would have my usual motion sickness, and I wasn't sure how I would react to the airport and airplane lighting. I knew I had to get help for myself, and I knew I had to do that now.

I was nervous heading off to Michigan. Thinking realistically I didn't want to get my hopes up too high, but in my heart I was more hopeful than I'd admitted. I'd reviewed the Vision Specialists website and saw that Dr. Debby had been practicing in this area for many years and that she really seemed to be quite knowledgeable about it, so I allowed myself to have hope. Although I was still a bit anxious, my husband and I were both excited and looking forward to it.

During my initial appointment, it was kind of strange wearing the prism test glasses and walking around the office, because my depth perception was now immediately improved and I wasn't yet used to that! Also, being able to see objects in my peripheral vision without having to actually turn first to see them was new to me. As a result, my neck was not straining from having to turn so often, eliminating that pain for me.

When flying back to California, after I got my prism glasses, I noticed that I didn't experience motion sickness at all! I used to have motion sickness every day. This felt totally different for me. It was hard for me to believe (and unless I'd experienced it, I would have found it very hard to accept) that by getting these kind of glasses my motion sickness could be eliminated.

My prism glasses have helped tremendously with the eye-strain issue I had. I can read longer without having to turn my head a lot, and working on the computer is effortless as I no longer get soreness in my eyes with that activity.

Prior to getting my prism glasses, I used to drive over curbs often. I used to tilt my head to one side, and I had to constantly turn my head to get the full view of the road. I felt like I had a permanent blind spot while driving. Instead of being able to just shift my eyes across the lanes of traffic, I had to turn my head all the time to look at the side-view mirrors, look in the rear-view mirror and then back to the road. My neck would get sore and I would feel exhausted, and that made me even more anxious. I'd be a nervous wreck by the time I'd gotten to where I was going.

I want to share my story with others who are also searching for answers and who may not have optometrists or physicians locally that are knowledgeable in the field of Vertical Heterophoria. Part of my mission in sharing my story is to get optometrists and others in the healthcare field interested in this study, so that people who are far from Michigan can seek help closer to home. Vision Specialists is wonderful at what they do, but realistically they can only see so many patients. It would be great for this information to become more wide spread, with other optometrists being trained in this field so that even more patients can be treated.

Since receiving my prism glasses, I no longer experience that daily motion sickness and I do not have the neck pain associated with the strain of having to turn my head often. In fact, I was talking with my mom after having received the prism glasses, and I told her I couldn't believe how much clarity I received with them, and that I was surprised to learn that other people have always had clarity. All this time I'd thought that everyone else was experiencing the same symptoms that I had, and I was amazed to find out that they weren't. I thought to myself: *'Wow! I never knew that people could feel this great everyday!'*

Part Four

Stories Of Those Who Have Dizziness And / Or Headache As Their Major Symptom(s)

I Don't Need A Wheelchair Anymore – I Can Walk Again!

by David McClellan

My story began in November, 2011. For some unknown reason, I became nauseated and started rapidly losing weight. Eventually I lost 25 pounds and I didn't know what was wrong. I wasn't able to keep food of any kind down. I also had no sense of balance, and was experiencing dizziness and was falling on a daily basis. If I bent over to pick something up I'd fall, and at times seemed about to pass out. Prior to these symptoms (that seemingly materialized out of nowhere) I was a very active, independent person.

Concerned about my health, my two daughters began taking me to various specialists to determine what was wrong and what could be done about it. For the next few months I had all kinds of tests run, but no answers were forthcoming. I had MRI's and X-Rays taken, I saw a neurologist, and even had some hospital stays, but no one knew what was wrong or what to do to alleviate my symptoms. I thought I'd had a mild stroke or something of that nature, but the test results dispelled that theory. As my ability to get around independently deteriorated, I became a resident of a nursing home, and for a month, was not able to get out of bed. During that difficult time, I wasn't able to receive rehabilitation activities or anything.

One day one of my daughters attended a sporting event for one of the local schools. A parent there asked her why I was no longer attending events. People were used to seeing me at the games because in the past I'd coached the younger students in softball. My daughter began to explain the unusual symptoms I'd been experiencing, and this parent happened to tell my daughter that my symptoms sounded similar to those of one of her cousins who had been able to find some answers and had been helped tremendously. She asked if she could have her cousin give us a call with more information. When her cousin called, she explained how she'd begun experiencing the same symptoms I had, and how at first, she thought she'd suffered a mild stroke as well. She'd gone to many specialists initially, and like me no one had a clue what was wrong or how to help her. Eventually someone told her about Vision Specialists of Michigan and suggested she give them a call. She said it was one of the best calls she'd ever made.

We gathered information from her about Vision Specialists of Michigan and my daughters checked out their website. Both my daughters became so   excited about what they read and how it related to my condition that together we completed the questionnaire and submitted it to Vision Specialists of Michigan. It wasn't long before we were contacted and an appointment was scheduled for me to be examined.

By this time I was using a wheelchair to get around as I simply could not stand without becoming dizzy and losing my balance. My weight had dropped considerably and I was no longer independent. I was desperate to receive legitimate help. I had no idea of just how much of my life would be given back to me as a result of making that appointment, but I was willing to see if Vision Specialists might have a viable solution for me.

Both my daughters went to the appointment with me. Dr. Debby conducted a very thorough eye examination. She asked many questions about what I'd been going through, when the symptoms first began and how I felt in relation to each symptom. She explained what prism glasses were and the many ways they might be able to benefit me. She also talked with me about Vertical

Heterophoria and how my eyes were misaligned, which contributed to many of the symptoms I now had.

After the examination, she placed a pair of the prism test glasses on me as I sat in my chair. I immediately had a clarity that I hadn't had before. Then she said to me: "Stand up. Place your feet solidly underneath you so that you feel good about the process, and start to walk towards me." At this point both my daughters jumped up and raced to my side, as they feared I might fall or quickly lose my balance because every time I'd attempted to walk previously I'd fallen over. I was nervous about trying to stand and walk without assistance, but Dr. Debby had been so confident and sure of herself when she asked me to do it that she made me feel confident in trying. When I hesitated for a moment, Dr. Debby smiled and said: "You'll be fine. You're able to do it." *Lifting myself from the chair was amazing!* To our surprise I walked all over her office! Then Dr. Debby took me outside and asked me to walk around freely. It was simply amazing. Both of my daughters cried right there in the office that day!

Initially I didn't have any expectations about going to Vision Specialist of Michigan. I'd never heard of Vertical Heterophoria or its' symptoms. I did not know anything about the information which the website contained, and I didn't have a clue about prism glasses or what their impact on my life could be. I was simply at a point where my overall general health had deteriorated so quickly and we did not have any answers as to what could possibly be wrong, even with all the specialists I'd been to and all of the various tests I'd taken. While it made sense to explore a different avenue, it didn't seem possible that all of what I'd experienced in the past several months could be connected to my eyes. But at this point I was ready to try anything, and exploring a different avenue made sense.

After I returned to the nursing home, the staff there was amazed. They couldn't believe their eyes, as I was able to be independent again – I could get out of bed and walk (sometimes with just the aid of a walker). I was no longer in a wheelchair! Eventually I was able to eliminate the walker and have been able to get back to my normal living again.

When I had my appointment with my family doctor, he too was amazed at the difference the prism glasses had made for me. He wasn't familiar with Vertical Heterophoria, so I was able to excitedly share information with him.

Since I've been wearing my prism glasses I'm able to read again (which I wasn't able to do because the words seemed to run together on the page). I no longer experience any dizziness, and I have my self-confidence and independence back. More importantly, I am now getting around without a wheelchair or the aid of a walker, and I am no longer living in a nursing home! I've been staying with one of my daughters as I recover, with plans to return to my own home soon. My entire life has been definitely changed!

Daughter Diana's Input: I had planned to shop with my dad one day, but as we were about to go into a store, he said he'd gotten awfully dizzy and wouldn't be able to go inside. He'd been feeling dizzy on and off for a short while, and although we were worried about him, this wasn't unusual, so we dropped him off at home for him to rest. I knew he was scheduled for a doctors' appointment in a few days, and we were looking forward to that. On the day of his appointment I received a call from his doctors' office advising me that my dad had missed his appointment. I immediately called his home and cell phone and did not get an answer. I have an aunt that lives near my dad, and I called her to ask if one of her sons would be able to go to check on him. When my cousin checked on him, he called to tell me that my dad hadn't been able to get out of bed for the last few days. I brought my dad to my home and immediately took him to a hospital to be examined, as he wasn't able to keep anything down, not even water. At first they thought it was gastroparesis because my dad is diabetic. They began treating him for that, but he didn't get any better and was still having to go back and forth for hospital stays as his condition worsened. He began falling often, and I was really afraid he would incur a major injury as a result. He began having physical therapy on a regular basis in an effort to improve his condition. I thought perhaps he'd experienced a stroke, as his motor skills were all askew and he couldn't seem to maintain his balance for any length of time. But all of the tests that were done showed no signs of a stroke or heart attack, so this all became even more mysterious to us.

The physical therapy was stopped when it was evident that my dads' condition was not improving, and he'd reached the point where he would literally be in the bed all day at the nursing home. He had to have someone assist him to go to the restroom - otherwise he would fall. These were major changes for him, as he'd been completely independent before.

To say that my sister and I were excited after reviewing the Vision Specialists of Michigan's website is putting it mildly. We were beside ourselves the more we read and the more we could see so many of the symptoms that my dad had been exhibiting over the months displayed on the site. It was uncanny. We helped him to complete the survey and anxiously waited to hear back with the results. We didn't have to wait long. Dr. Debby called and talked with us, and then we set up an appointment to have Dad seen.

My sister and I accompanied Dad to his appointment at Vision Specialists of Michigan. We weren't sure just what the possibilities for change would be, but we were sure hoping we'd finally receive some answers and some information as to what our next steps would be. The entire staff was genuinely concerned about being able to assist us in finding answers, and they went out of the way to make us all feel really comfortable.

When Dr. Debby first instructed my dad to get up and walk across the room towards her while wearing the test prism glasses, my sister and I bolted from where we sat to rush to his side, but Dr. Debby said: "No, he'll be fine. He can do it." When he actually did it, we both burst into tears. It was simply unbelievable! Especially when you consider how he hadn't been able to walk unassisted for some time. She then took him out to the waiting room area to walk around for a few moments before having us all go outside to have him walk there as well. I simply couldn't believe what I was witnessing. I nervously waited for him to fall or lose his balance, but he never did.

Even now, to see him back in his normal routine is indescribable. My sister and I were gung-ho to take him to this appointment because we were thinking we simply had nowhere else to turn. We never imagined the result would be that he'd be able to get out of his wheelchair and walk without falling. It truly seemed to be Divine Intervention that occurred for us. What other explanation is there for this situation? Out of the blue, this parent just happened to ask about my dad, and she immediately recognized that the symptoms her cousin had experienced were the same symptoms that my sister was describing that Dad was experiencing. We'd been to all kinds of specialists and my dad had undergone various tests and treatments but we weren't able to see any improvements at all. Meanwhile my dad's condition had deteriorated to the point where he was lying all day in a bed in a nursing home! He felt helpless. How frustrating that must have been for him. To then take him to an appointment to see an optometrist and within a few hours see him get up from a wheelchair and be able to walk - there is no greater feeling and no way to truly express it! My dad is now cooking and eating and has gotten back up to his normal weight. He's able to be independent again. He has stayed with me for about six weeks, just to ensure he's his usual self, and we're looking forward to his return to his own home. He has even been able to drive again (with some restrictions) and it's allowed him even more autonomy.

In conclusion, I'd like to say we had no idea that Vision Specialists of Michigan would be able to change our entire lives so completely. It didn't just impact my dad, but me and my sister as well. We weren't able to just identify my dad's ailment - we were able to obtain the cure!

I'm 200% Better And Can Smile And Laugh Again!

by Joann Gazal   *Story 27*

I've needed corrective lenses since 4th grade, so going for eye exams and wearing glasses was not an issue for me. However in my later years, there came a time when I went to pick up a new pair of prescription glasses and put them on, and thought: *'These can't be mine. I can't see a thing out of them.'* I told my eye doctor and he examined me again, and stated that my eyes had changed drastically since the 10 days prior when I'd been in to have them checked! One would think it was a fluke of some sort, or perhaps the calibrations of the machines were askew in some way, but believe it or not, this actually happened with me three times in a row. I'd have my eyes examined thoroughly and afterwards I'd go in to pick up the glasses only to realize the prescription was as if it'd been written for someone else! Can you imagine having your eye doctor tell you within a 10 day time frame: "These glasses aren't for you now, but they *were* for you - 10 days ago!" As a result, I was sent to a specialist at a local hospital eye center.

It just so happens that I'd been having other issues as well. I'd get really sick when driving, and had begun to have really bad headaches. I'd become physically ill if I had to look to my left or turn my head in that direction at all. So driving would almost be comical, as I'd gotten to the point where I had to make all right turns, which sometimes resulted in my actually going five miles out of the way—just to get to my desired destination while avoiding turning left! Of course looking back, I can see how ridiculous my life had become, but we do what we have to do on a daily basis to cope with the situation at hand. I'd reasoned that it hadn't always been this way for me and had convinced myself that this too shall pass, but as the years went by my symptoms became more pronounced and more noticeable and were affecting other areas of my daily life.

To make matters worse, while trying to get a handle on why I was having these symptoms, I'd begun suffering from a severe case of vertigo and was preparing to have ear surgery. My vertigo had escalated to the point where I couldn't stand up properly and I couldn't look down without feeling faint or dizzy. It was horrible!

Unfortunately, after the surgery my symptoms didn't go away, and while conducting a post-surgery examination, it was my ear doctor that advised me that my symptoms had nothing to do with my ears. He then referred me to Dr. Debby at Vision Specialists. He explained that he'd attended a seminar about the work that Dr. Debby and the staff at Vision Specialists were doing with prism lenses and Vertical Heterophoria, and he thought it might be the remedy for me.

By the time he'd referred me to Dr. Debby, I was seriously ready to discover what was going on with me and get it fixed. I reluctantly had to take a medical leave from work for five months while trying to find out what was causing my symptoms and what could be done about my eyes. I was willing to try anything. I'd never heard of prism glasses, so I wasn't that optimistic that they would make a difference for me. I had reached a point where I thought: *'Oh God, nothing can help me.'* But I was just fed up with not feeling well, and was willing to give them a try.

During my initial examination, with the questions that Dr. Debby posed to me, it became clear that I'd overlooked many symptoms from as far back as my early youth. There were seemingly small things that I hadn't paid any attention to that now garnered my attention. Like my having motion sickness when I'd go up a small hill or incline. All my sisters would be fine, but I would go: 'Whoa!' It just didn't feel like a normal experience for me. I'd also discounted my head tilt. I'd tilted my head towards my right side for years, and never gave it a second thought.

It turns out I needed to have the vertical as well as the horizontal prisms for my glasses. In my particular case, I was able to understand that my eyes had been struggling with Vertical Heterophoria for years and it was as if they had finally declared: *'We're tired. We are tired of fighting vertically and horizontally and we don't have the strength to continue in this way.'*

Believe me, the time off for medical leave was well worth it to get my prism glasses! Had I not fully taken care of this issue when I did, I'm convinced I would not have been able to continue to drive, and as a result, would not have been able to return to my employment. Prior to getting my prism glasses, whenever I drove, it was like wearing blinders. I could see everything directly in front of me, but I wasn't able to see things around me.

As with any pair of new glasses there's a period of adjustment, but there's a difference between going through a period of adjustment, and knowing when you've finally found the solution. And that difference is freeing! With the prism glasses, my headaches went away. The buzzing in my ears went away. The vertigo has been greatly reduced. I have clarity in my vision and am able to read much more comfortably than I did before. I used to experience blurred vision and the lines on the pages would appear to run together as if the sentences were all moving. Right now, I can tell you that I am 200% better than I was initially. *My life is totally different. I'm able to smile and laugh again!*

What I'd like people to understand is that depending on your symptoms, how long you've been experiencing them and to what degree, it may take a few appointments before your particular prism prescription is determined, but rest assured that the entire staff at Vision Specialists will work really well with you, and will be very patient and will do what it takes to diagnose and fit you with the correct prescription.

My goal is to spread the word to as many people as I can, about Vision Specialists and the work they do. It's really important for you to know that you might be experiencing symptoms in a part of your body that you think has nothing to do with your eyes, and yet it could be visually mediated. The list of VH symptoms on the website can help you figure this out.

Ultimately the ear doctor who referred me to Vision Specialists took pictures of me in my new glasses to show other patients when he refers them to their office. It gives him the opportunity to share with them my story about how the prism glasses have made a big difference for me in my life. The good thing is that we are blessed with the technology we have now, so that children and adults are able to take advantage of the years of research and hard work that Vision Specialists has done, that simply wasn't available years ago.

I'm indebted to Vision Specialists for all of the hard work they did to help me improve. For anyone out there who is experiencing the symptoms that Vision Specialists has on their web site, your gift to yourself should be to fill out the on-line survey to see if you might benefit from prism glasses.

I Was So Sick From VH, I Just Wanted To Die – And Almost Chose To Do So

by Dr. L. L. *Story 28*

About 12 years ago, I started suffering from severe dizziness. Not the kind of dizziness that most people associate with vertigo, but a different kind - one that was hard to explain. I also noticed I'd get headaches that were very painful and take a while to go away. My eyes started to hurt a lot, and I went to optometrists and ophthalmologists to determine what was going on. However, the regular eye exams weren't able to diagnose or pin-point the cause of the eye pain. I tried to cope with these symptoms as best I could. At times, I'd treat myself with herbal medicines (which seemed to help) but I still needed to find out what was causing my problems.

Gradually my symptoms worsened. At times my headaches would be so excruciating that I could not open my eyes without experiencing extreme pain. Imagine having a condition where it is too painful to even open your eyes! I had developed a disturbing ringing in my left ear, which made it difficult to hear others when they spoke. In efforts to quiet the ringing and to focus my vision, I'd begun tilting my head to one side, which caused severe neck pain. Due to my feelings of dizziness and imbalance, I'd become afraid of using the staircase and would look for an elevator instead. Soon, even driving became difficult to do.

In our search for answers, my husband and I began to wonder if perhaps I might have a brain tumor. I had CT scans, X-Rays, MRI's and a series of other tests, but they all came back normal. There was no answer as to why I was experiencing such varied and seemingly unrelated symptoms.

I then began to experience feelings of anxiety and paranoia. I'd never before in my life experienced these symptoms - they made no sense whatsoever to me. I began to wonder if I was bi-polar, or maybe I was just going through some sort of psychological episode. Regardless, I had difficulty functioning normally.

I had also developed difficulty with depth perception. As a dentist, this kept me from being able to focus on my patients properly - their noses seemed to now protrude from their faces in a strange way. I was afraid of making errors. Noises had become distracting to me, and I found it hard to deal with even the soft music playing in the background of the patients' rooms.

When I returned home after a long day's work, I would be cranky and irritable from trying to cope with these unusual symptoms. Sadly, I realized my symptoms were now taking up a very large part of my life. Even my performance as a mother was being affected - I was frequently pushing my two young sons away from me in my effort to relax and unwind. I was always feeling anxious, and I realized I was no longer able to concentrate fully at home or at work. I had no one to talk to about any of this, and felt I had nowhere to turn. All the while, doctors were not able to determine the cause of any of these symptoms, and some doctors were even telling me it was all 'in my head'. I'd begun to think that my sons and my husband deserved much more than I was able to give to them, and thought how their lives would be dramatically improved if I simply weren't around anymore. At my lowest point, I began having suicidal thoughts - I had developed a very brutal plan to kill myself. I didn't like having these thoughts and tried desperately not to entertain them, but as time passed and my desperation increased, these types of thoughts became frequent.

While searching on-line for answers, my husband happened to come across a website forum that talked about many of the symptoms I'd been experiencing, and one of the participants had listed information about the Vision Specialists of Michigan's website. We reviewed that website and were amazed that all of the symptoms listed for a vision condition called Vertical Heterophoria (VH) matched what I'd been experiencing!

That website was a God-send. It was very easy to read, and I knew within just a few minutes that I most likely had VH. I was interested in finding out more, so I clicked on the link and filled out the questionnaire to see if I might have VH. The questions contained in the questionnaire addressed so many of my symptoms that I really felt hopeful. I was surprised that I got a call back, that it happened so quickly, and that it was from Dr. Debby herself. She discussed the questionnaire results with me, and thought that I could benefit from an evaluation. I was so desperate by this point (I had been seen by so many different doctors, had tried so many different remedies that did not work, and had even been to the emergency room twice) that I was willing to try anything with even the slightest chance of helping me obtain relief.

I'd worn glasses since I was 12 years old, so I was familiar with getting my eyes examined, and I can say with some authority that the eye exam at Vision Specialists of Michigan was unlike any eye exam I had experienced in the past - it was so much more thorough and complete. Dr. Debby asks questions specifically related to your symptoms that were discovered in the questionnaire you completed, and she performs an examination personally tailored to suit your vision needs. For patients with VH, a cookie-cutter eye exam simply will not do.

The first time I tried on the prism test glasses and stood up, I felt as if I'd been stretched out, but in a good way. I was able to stand taller and straighter and walk with more ease and confidence, whereas before, my body felt like an accordion, wound tight and tense. Another very clear sign for me was that my tinnitus went away - no more ear ringing for me! I also soon noticed that I had no more neck pain - *it was simply gone*. Over time, I realized I was no longer afraid of taking the stairs; and without feeling imbalanced, my gait and my stance improved. Also, my stress and anxiety improved markedly, and my suicidal thoughts ceased.

My reason for sharing my story is to let as many people as possible (from educators in schools and Universities to those working in organizations and corporations and in the medical community) know that there are *millions* who are currently suffering from VH and who have no idea that a simple set of prism lenses could heal them. Just think about it: If you could eliminate excruciating migraines, blurred or double vision, sensitivity to light, feelings of anxiety, the fear of going to shopping malls or being in open public spaces, and difficulty with reading with a simple pair of prism lenses, wouldn't you? Just think of all of the tests, procedures, and therapies that could be avoided, and all of the money that could be saved!

Just one example of the hidden nature of VH: If children are having difficulty with reading, or have a tendency to 'skip lines', it is possible that VH might be the culprit. Children who are struggling and falling behind in school will most likely be unable to articulate or communicate how they're feeling. Unless they are asked specific questions about the symptoms of VH, they will never be diagnosed and will continue to struggle needlessly.

The problem is, many of the symptoms of VH aren't classically thought to be vision or eye-related at all, and that is why the connection doesn't get made - even amongst professionals in the medical community.

I am so happy to be a part of the book project because it's important to me that people know about VH. I truly thought I was going crazy and that there was no help for me out there. I almost died from this condition. Thank goodness my husband found out about VH and Vision Specialists, and that we were able to travel to Michigan to obtain treatment. However, it shouldn't have to be so difficult to be diagnosed and treated for VH. There needs to be a major education effort for medical personnel so that they can recognize VH in their patients, along with training a cadre of optometrists located throughout the country to care for these patients. I hope this happens soon, for the sake of all of those who are suffering.

Prism Glasses Have Helped My Marriage

by Carolyn Monaco   *Story 29*

The symptom that got me to Dr. Debby at Vision Specialists was headaches. I had terrible headaches every day and at times they'd become excruciating. My mom and sister used to get migraines, so of course I thought that was just the way it was. I was prescribed a medication for the migraines, and when it would get really bad, I'd use it.

I'd experienced these headaches since high school but the headaches weren't a major issue for me until I got into my thirties

On one particular day, I'd gotten a migraine that was simply unbearable. I was at the point where I was willing to put my head through a wall in order to knock myself out - that's literally how bad it felt. I decided to go to the emergency room. Coincidentally, Dr. Debby's husband was the attending emergency physician and he noticed the way I was tilting my head. He asked me some questions about other symptoms, many of which I had. He thought I might have a condition called Vertical Heterophoria. He explained that I might be a candidate for glasses with prism in them. He went on to say that the major problems I'd been experiencing for so long might stem from this eye condition.

To be honest, I was very skeptical initially because he also explained that his wife, Dr. Debby, was the doctor spearheading this research. I thought: *"I'm being had. He is recommending his wife (who is an optometrist) just to give her business."* But my husband encouraged me by reminding me of how bad my headaches get and he asked: ***"What do you have to lose to at least check it out? If anything can help you with those darned***

headaches then you should be willing to at least go to hear what they have to say. " Little did I know, my husband was also tired of all of the limitations placed on me because of my headaches, and he desperately wanted me to get better.

My husband accompanied me to the first appointment and let me tell you, it was more than just an eye appointment for me. It was a very emotional experience. I'd had no idea how much your eyes can affect other areas of your health and affect how you feel overall. I just cried after Dr. Debby fitted me with prisms for the first time. I learned more about Vertical Heterophoria, and was able to understand that for years my eye muscles had been straining to keep my eyes aligned and to prevent double vision. I'd simply reached a point where my eye muscles didn't have the strength to continue that battle. As a result, I began to tilt my head in order to help keep the images aligned and to see clearly, which caused my neck pain. Since my eye muscles were struggling constantly, I began experiencing terrible migraines, which eventually led to my going to the emergency room for some relief (if only temporary).

Amazingly now, as soon as I begin having headaches, I know I have to have an appointment to have my prescription updated, because that's my first clue that my eye muscles are being overused and need the assistance of the correct prism to stay on track. Like any other vision prescription, our eyes change over time and adjustments are needed.

Since being diagnosed with Vertical Heterophoria and receiving prism glasses, my social life has changed dramatically! Before getting the prism glasses, I'd get out of work or school and I'd be totally exhausted. My head would hurt, my eyes would hurt, and all I wanted to do was go straight home. My husband wanted to go out and do things, but I just couldn't. Trying to see a movie was horrendous. I'd go with my husband and he'd get very upset with me because if we went to an action movie, the constant movement on the screen would make me so nauseous that I'd get physically sick. I'd explain to him that I couldn't stay and we'd have to leave and we'd just fight on the way back home about it. He simply didn't understand how watching a movie could make me sick, and frankly I didn't understand it either, and I didn't know how to convey that to him. Looking back on it all, I can see how he must have felt, thinking I just didn't want to see the particular movie he'd chosen, but that wasn't it at all.

Before getting the prism glasses, I had a number of problems. When driving, I'd run over things all the time. I was unable to avoid pot-holes in the road. I was driving too close to the curb. If I saw something in the road and moved to avoid it, I'd hit it anyway. I didn't have the peripheral vision - I'd actually have to turn my head and focus directly on what I was looking at in order to see objects clearly. Constantly turning my head left and right while driving just made my neck pain worse, but it was something I told myself I had to deal with. I was getting nauseous bending down and looking back up, which normally people take for granted and do without thinking about it. It was just a horrible feeling. And most people just don't understand what it is like having to deal with all of this on a daily basis.

Since having my prism glasses, the motion sickness has stopped and my peripheral vision has improved. But the number one improvement as far as I'm concerned is that my headaches - those excruciating, terrible headaches have stopped! All of these symptoms improved very quickly after I started wearing the prism glasses. It was simply amazing!

The changes from wearing the prism glasses go well beyond just 'being able to see more clearly,' – my entire personality was affected. I became more confident, and as a result, more outgoing. I was able to begin enjoying a social life by going out with colleagues after work and not having to just go straight home. Before, I'd just thought of myself as a sickly person who was no fun to be around. I just felt bad about myself. But that all changed after getting these prism glasses. Additionally, it was good that my husband was at my appointment to find out that I actually had a condition that caused the headaches, the motion sickness and the nausea when watching movies. It was such an emotionally freeing experience for him to finally understand that I wasn't 'just making it all up to avoid social situations.' It was a huge relief for the both of us. He used to tell me it was all in my head, and he'd get angry and say that I just wasn't trying hard enough to be social or go with the flow. Finding out that there was a cause for all of these symptoms was vindicating for me.

What are the odds of my having gone to the emergency room, and having the emergency physician notice my symptoms, recommend me to his optometrist-wife, overcome my skepticism to go see her, and have all of these issues resolve for me? That's not going to happen with everyone. That's why I wanted to share this story. People who are suffering through life with head tilts, neck pain, vertigo, awful headaches or motion sickness really need to learn about Vertical Heterophoria and whether they, too, may be candidates for prism glasses. In addition, eye doctors need training so that they can correctly diagnose and treat VH, and help all of those people who have VH get relief from their symptoms.

Lastly, I wanted to share information about my father. My father was a lawyer. He was sick all the time with nausea. He never wanted to go out and became very reclusive. Even as a lawyer, he wasn't very confident and it's easy for me to see now that he suffered from some of the same symptoms that I had. I really feel that it was all related to his eyes as well. Can you imagine what his life could have been like had he had the opportunity when he was younger to be diagnosed and treated for VH? His way of life would have been completely different. My life would have also been different if I had received treatment earlier in my own life. I can tell you my college years would have definitely been different. I wanted to go into advertising and marketing but because of my symptoms I was just too shy and simply could not do it. It was just too overwhelming and I just wanted to go and be someplace quiet. Looking back, and being honest, even my marriage would have been different.

Before getting my prism glasses, I was always telling my husband: "I don't want to do that because it makes me nauseous, I can't go to movies or I'd get sick" or "I just want to go home and be still." When you're with someone that is constantly shutting down any kind of social life, it has to be challenging for the spouse to deal with over the years. It leaves you mourning the kind of life you could have had.

I feel so blessed to be one of the many patients of Vision Specialists, and to have been helped so tremendously.

Now when people tell me they've always had headaches, I immediately tell them to go and get their eyes checked. They tell me how they don't think the two conditions are related and I tell them how I didn't think so either prior to getting my prism glasses. And that's understandable, because when you hear the word 'headache' you think 'head,' not eyes. We neglect to remember that our eyes are in our heads! And there is just so much information that needs to be out there in relation to this.

I really wish my dad could be alive to see and know about this information. Even better if he'd have had the opportunity to experience the impact it could've made for him. Believe me, it makes a major difference in your life when you can get up and not feel bad everyday.

Valium and Vodka Helped Me Cope Until I Was Cured By Prism Glasses

by Yolanda Wright   *Story 30*

Prior to learning about Vision Specialists and getting my prism glasses, the symptoms I experienced for many years were a total mystery to not only me, but to the medical community as well. For that reason, I referred to my symptoms as the 'Silent Disability.' But allow me to explain:

To begin with, my case was a long one. Reflecting back on it all, I can say I began to realize the full brunt of what was happening to me when I was about 28 years old. I'd been attending beauty school for about 6 months, and while putting a customer under the dryer, all of a sudden it felt as if someone were pushing me to the ground. I started to shake uncontrollably but somehow managed to get the customer under the dryer before making my way to the nearest chair and sitting down. My instructor came to my side and I explained that I thought I was about to pass out. I became very dizzy, but it was more than just that. It's the kind of feeling you get when you're seated in your car in a parking lot, and the car next to you begins to pull out, and for a split-second you can't tell if it's your car that is moving or if it's the other car. You panic as you try to get your bearings and determine what's really happening. My husband had to come to the beauty school to pick me up that day. I was too dizzy and disoriented to go home alone.

Other symptoms began to plague me. When going shopping, the lights in the stores seemed to be too bright. I realized my eyes were very sensitive to light - especially the bright lights like the kind you experience outside of your home. I tried to finish beauty school (as I didn't have many more months to go in order to complete the training) but it became a problem because I started having dizzy spells when driving. Also, upon arriving at the school, the thought of taking a customer would send me into a kind of panic mode. Not knowing when I might experience dizziness made me anxious. I was able to confide in my instructor, and by working within the new limitations that I was now experiencing, she adjusted my schedule and duties so that I could finish the course. She was such a wonderful blessing for me at that time, and I was able to complete my final exam and pass the course with a lot of concentrated effort and work.

But my symptoms didn't go away. Shopping became worse as the sensitivity to the bright lights made my eyes hurt and gave me headaches. In addition to that, the everyday noises of shopping were magnified to me. A simple shopping cart slightly hitting another one accidentally, or a door opening and shutting seemed to be too loud for me to bear.

My house became my refuge. I no longer wanted to go out, but I had to learn how to deal with the task of everyday living. I had to give up grocery shopping and driving. Because of this, I opened a beauty shop in my home. I thought having the customers come to me would be the solution to my being unable to travel. However this did not resolve my other symptoms, and with my second customer I began to shake uncontrollably again. My solution to that was to run upstairs to get a shot of alcohol so that I could finish working with my customer in a more relaxed state. In the meantime, I started going to different types of doctors to find out what was going on with me physically, and what could be done to correct it.

Without knowing what was going on, I was convinced that I was dying. As a result, I had a family photo taken so that my children would have it after I was gone. As the years progressed, with different medical professionals telling me they weren't sure what was wrong, and with the symptoms I was experiencing having come from out of nowhere, I'd come to the conclusion that 'this was it and I'd may as well prepare for it staying like this.'

Doctors asked me if I'd ever experienced any of these symptoms. Looking back, I remembered an incident in school many years ago. I was in the 6th grade and used to love to read out loud. I was called upon to do so, and for some reason I couldn't do it. I became short of breath and panicked, unable to complete the task. After that, whenever I thought a teacher would call on me, I'd have a panic episode. From that time forward I avoided that type of situation at all costs. All the way through high school I was able to avoid public speaking. However, there was a mandatory event I wasn't going to be able to escape. In order to graduate high school, each student had to give a short speech. During my senior year I made friends with a girl whose mother wanted her to go to a finishing school in a different state. This is a type of school that prepared women to have careers outside of the home, like becoming a secretary or personal assistant. My friend did not want to go alone and invited me to accompany her. My first thought was: '*I could go and not have to worry about doing a speech in front of a group of people in order to graduate.*' So the next week we were on our way to finishing school together. I completed the finishing schools' requirements and was able to secure a job as a typist at a bank, and I was relieved that I never had to give that mandatory speech in order to graduate high school.

Some of the doctors I consulted with for relief of my symptoms felt that the problems I was experiencing were solely mental rather than physical. My symptoms (which included dizziness, headaches, sensitivity to lights, vertigo, and mild instances of agoraphobia) had begun to disable me in such a significant manner that I began to read self-help books and seek help from traditional as well as holistic health care professionals (including a hypnotist). None of these avenues helped, but I was not going to give up hope.

As time went on I found a new way of coping. I used my prescription Valium and combined it with alcohol. I wasn't too thrilled about coping in this way, but it helped me to get through the dizziness and be able to leave home without the anxiety attacks I was so prone to having. I told myself the alcohol was totally medicinal. But having alcohol on my breath on a daily basis began to weigh heavily on me. I had a strong sense of guilt, a lack of pride, and a low self-image - it just stripped me of everything I valued. I thought if I focused more on my children, I'd be able to cope better with my life.

One day I became aware that I was straining to see clearly and having double vision, and I realized there was something seriously wrong with my eyes. Even though I wore glasses at the time, I'd never heard of Vertical Heterophoria before, so I wasn't even aware that it could cause many of the symptoms that I'd been experiencing. While searching on my computer to find answers, I looked up information having to do with problems with eyes or eyesight. This was how I came upon the website for Vision Specialists. As I began to read the information there, I thought: '*I can't believe what I'm seeing!*' The information there described so many of the symptoms that I'd been experiencing for so many years that at first I thought it was some sort of a scam. But at that point I was ready to try anything to help me, so I contacted Dr. Debby, and after speaking with me for awhile she told me she had a questionnaire for me to complete to determine if I were a candidate for the prism glasses. After reviewing it, Dr. Debby called to let me know that my questionnaire score was high, that I might have Vertical Heterophoria, and that prism glasses might be of help to me.

After having spoken with her and understanding what she was explaining to me, I really hoped to go into her office and come out a different person. Even after having seen all of the other medical practitioners and having tried all of the different methods over the years, I knew in my heart my symptoms were not related to a mental illness (even though some doctors had tried to convince me of that since they had been unable to diagnose what was happening).

I can tell you I had never experienced the kind of eye exam that Dr. Debby performed during my visits to her. She fitted me with prism test glasses and sent me to the grocery store with my husband to see how I would feel with the new lenses. She also had me walk along the sidewalk in front of her office with the glasses on to see how comfortable I felt with them.

I want people to know that sometimes the very first visit may not alleviate all of your symptoms. My eyes and my symptoms did improve somewhat during the first visit, but it took a few more visits and exams before I was able to experience the marked improvements that I now have. At one point I had become discouraged and was ready to give up and quit, but Dr. Debby worked tirelessly with me and told me: "I'm not going to give up."

Shortly after that, I was out in my backyard wearing the prism glasses, and I thought to myself: *"Something's definitely different out here."* I looked around me and noticed that without straining at all, everything looked closer and sharper. I was so excited! Afterwards, I noticed two major improvements: While shopping, I noticed the bright lights in the stores weren't so daunting anymore and I was able to stand and talk to people without falling over or feeling unbalanced or getting that pitched forward feeling! And I remember thinking then, *"Wow, this isn't going to last, it must be a fluke."* But the longer I wore the glasses the more my symptoms improved. My improvements didn't happen right away, but the important thing is - they happened! I was so happy and felt like I could finally relax.

Now I feel like I'm a totally new person. I have my life back on track again. I am now able to drive, I can go out again, and I'm able to see clearly and read without difficulty. I've even been able to get on a plane and fly to California to see my daughter! I wasn't able to do that before because of the anxiety I felt while just waiting in the airport. My daughter was absolutely thrilled for me.

When I returned home, I mentioned to my doctor I was able to board a plane and fly, and he asked for Dr. Debby's card from me, so that he could refer other patients that may be candidates for the prism glasses!

I am totally flabbergasted with all of the improvements I've been able to experience, and I try to tell everyone I know to check out Vision Specialists and the work that the entire staff does for its patients. You don't have to suffer through years of debilitating, limiting symptoms, and you don't have to develop coping mechanisms to get you through them. If there's a chance you or someone you know might be a candidate for prism glasses, go and get more information from their website, or talk with the wonderful staff of Vision Specialists.

Lab Coat With Wings

by Vickie Schweller

It's hard for me to tell my story, simply because of all the time, pain, discomfort, aggravation and everything that it caused me. For a while, I was a prisoner in my own home.

My story starts in January, 2010. Prior to that, I'd been relatively healthy all of my life. I had never experienced any of the symptoms (which I'm about to share with you) that happened to me for a period of 15 months. It was unclear why all of a sudden this was happening - the whole experience was quite a mystery to me.

One day, for reasons unknown to me, I began experiencing continuous vertigo, migraines and double and blurred vision. My dizziness and migraines were so acute, that I could not walk without holding onto the walls or furniture. I could no longer drive, walk my dog, or even take the one step down from my kitchen to my garage without falling and injuring myself.

My independent lifestyle was shattered, as I even had to have help in and out of the shower. I was unable to do anything on my own. To make matters worse, there was nothing that had occurred to me that caused these symptoms to begin. I hadn't taken a fall, I hadn't been involved in any car accidents, and I hadn't fainted prior to experiencing these symptoms.

It was too frustrating and embarrassing to go out in public. My muscle tone was gone and I had no strength of my own. My husband was now relegated to going to work and coming home to take care of me and everything else. He never complained and he was my biggest supporter. When my family would take me out, I had to have assistance to get in and out of the car, be helped into the restaurant and to my seat. I became very self-conscious and felt that people would think I was drunk. That became a good reason for me to not go out anymore. I told my husband I should design a T-shirt that reads: *'I'm not drunk—it's just vertigo.'*

I began to isolate myself. I could not turn the stove on, as I was afraid I might pass out and the stove or oven would still be on for hours before it would be discovered. I refused to accept assistance from well-meaning friends who offered to help with chores around the house, or who wanted to bring meals for me and my husband. Soon, I stopped taking their phone calls altogether. I didn't want anyone to witness how debilitated and limited my life had become. I just stopped living. I existed—and that was it.

I missed out on a great deal of my life and events that were very important to me. I missed my grandson's birthday dinner and all of his sports events. I missed seeing my granddaughter off to her prom and taking pictures with her. I missed school and church events, and I even missed being able to visit with my terminally ill grandson. I was unable to be in the 4th of July parade (which I hadn't missed since 1991). I was no longer able to volunteer to help our troops and veterans, which were programs that I spear-headed in our community for Desert Storm and Desert Shield. I was not able to attend weddings, funerals, holiday get-togethers, pancake breakfasts, Mother's Day dinners, and the Memorial for families of Flight 93 in Pennsylvania (which you may recall, was one of the hijacked planes that crashed on 9/11). My grandchildren were not able to come over to spend nights with me because I couldn't cook for them, tuck them in, read a story to them, or do any of the things grandparents normally do during overnight stays.

This lifestyle was very hard to deal with mentally, physically and financially. It took its' toll on all aspects of my living. I kept wondering why this happened to me, and what could be done about it. I went to a neurologist and he prescribed various medications, but none of them worked. It was suggested that I go to an ENT (Ear/Nose/Throat) specialist. I went there and he wasn't able to find anything. I had numerous tests done from one health care professional to another, with no results. I was sent to specialty clinics for more tests, and still nothing. I worked with physical therapists for a time, but unfortunately that did not yield any results. I began to think that I may have a brain tumor or that I was just dying from some unknown cause. There were times when I thought I'd be better off dying, as I was putting so much of a burden on my husband now, and I didn't feel it was fair to him. I wanted to have a good quality of life and not just a life, and until you experience what that means for you personally, it's hard to understand. I was at the point where I could no longer even read. And I'd loved reading!

I was told at one point that I would just have to sit all day, to avoid falling. I thought to myself; *how can anyone just sit? Especially someone that had been as active as I'd always been?* I tried it, but I would look at my home and become depressed at all that needed to be done that I could no longer do. I would see the dust under the table that needed to be tended to; I longed to be able to cook dinner; but I'd tell myself I was to simply follow instructions and just sit. You can only watch TV so much, and it was just mind-boggling for me. I was reminded of the cartoon character that gets hit on the head and you see the little birdies flying around their head, that's the way I felt. When I tried to read it was painful, as it felt like my eyes were going around and around in my head. I felt terrible.

My husband couldn't take time off from work everyday, and with my not being able to drive, I couldn't do even simple tasks anymore, like going to get a mammogram, going to the dentist, going grocery shopping or taking the dog to the vet. For my really important appointments my husband would have to take time from work to assist me in getting those things done. I had to wait for him to come home to cook and I could not even load or unload the dishwasher, because bending would cause me to get dizzy and fall.

In an effort to find relief, I went back to the neurologist and asked what else could be done. He recommended another clinic that specialized in some of the symptoms I was having, and so away we went. I had blood work done and an assessment to see if I would be a candidate for the hospital. It turns out I was a candidate, and was admitted as a patient for 15 days. But the methods they tried did not work for me. They tried a number of different medications to see what might work. I left there with many medications and yet I still was not well.

Ironically, the day I was being released from that hospital, someone had made an appointment for me at Vision Specialists with Dr. Debby. I'd never even heard of Dr. Debby or Vision Specialists, but by this time (as you can imagine) I was willing to try any reasonable recommendation that was given to me. Prior to going to see Dr. Debby for the first time, I did not have any expectations of being able to be relieved of any of my symptoms because by the time I was referred to her, I'd been going to specialists for 15 months with no relief. To me, going to see her was just another doctors' appointment.

Thankfully, this is where my story makes a complete turn-around. I went to my appointment with Dr. Debby and before she closed that night, I had a pair of the prism glasses. I put them on and immediately my vertigo went away! In fact, I have not had a migraine or experienced vertigo since that day!

Dr. Debby explained that I had Vertical Heterophoria, and that this was a condition I was quite possibly born with. She also explained that after years of my eyes and body straining to adapt, my eye muscles were now too fatigued to maintain the constant struggle, which may have caused the other symptoms to manifest. I'm over 60 years old. I'd worn eyeglasses since the 4th grade, yet not one eye doctor has ever mentioned this condition to me. I don't think they did so out of neglect. It's just that doctors are not trained in this area, and therefore do not know how to diagnose and treat it properly.

When I first tried on the prism test glasses, and stood to get out of the chair in the exam room, I literally felt like I was 10 feet tall. I'm just 5 foot even, but I felt so confident and so different! I actually had a bounce in my step when I walked and I didn't feel dizzy, woozy, nauseous, or any of that. The only thing I could compare it to was this: When I was a kid in grade school, my teacher sent me home with a note, advising that I may need glasses. My grandmother took me to the 2nd floor of this big bank building which was where the eye doctor's office was located and I got my first pair of eyeglasses. I stood at the top of those stairs to walk down and it was like: Oh my gosh, I could see everything! I could make everything out and it was like I was able to open my eyes for the first time. Getting the prism glasses was like that for me as well. It was as if I were finally able to really see clearly, for the very first time in my life. Over time, we get to a point in our lives where we adapt to our deficiencies and we think it's normal and ok and then we find out it's not.

My husband was elated! He couldn't believe it! All the way home from my first appointment we were so excited about the immediate change - to this day we don't take any of it for granted. Believe me, Dr. Debby has become a household word for us around here.

Dr. Debby and Vision Specialists are not only able to diagnose the problem of Vertical Heterophoria, they're also able to offer a solution for it. I do not blame the other specialists that I saw, or the ophthalmologists that I went to over the years, but it takes someone like Dr. Debby who is sincerely passionate about what she does, someone with such a loving heart that truly cares about their patients, in order to make the kind of difference that I was able to have. In fact, the entire staff of Vision Specialists exemplifies the very characteristics that Dr. Debby showcases. She has even called me at home on a Saturday to see how my eyeglasses are working for me and to ask if I'm having any problems.

Once when going to Dr. Debby for a routine eye exam, I was experiencing some neck and right shoulder pain. Dr. Debby saw how much pain I was in. She called a therapist that she knows and was able to get me in to see them the next day. She truly goes out of the way to get you help even in areas beyond just your eyes.

I'm so excited about the major positive changes I've been able to experience as a result of having gone to Vision Specialists that I've had their staff make me up two different kinds of folders with information about Vision Specialists and the important work they are doing for me to pass out to people. One folder is geared towards professionals in the medical field like other doctors and chiropractors, to help them recognize a patient that might benefit from what Vision Specialists does and refer them. The other folder is for patients that are experiencing some of the symptoms of Vertical Heterophoria. When I talk to them I hand a folder directly to them. I've given folders out to family, friends, neighbors and others. People need to know about this, especially anyone that has a problem with vertigo or dizziness.

Dr. Debby and the staff at Vision Specialists cared enough to find out about VH and study it, and educate themselves on how to fix it. They've done years of painstaking research as well as built upon the research and progress of doctors from the past, to help them better care for people with VH.

I refer to Dr. Debby as my 'lab coat with wings' because to me, she was my personal miracle worker. After years of not having answers, Dr. Debby was able to properly diagnose me within a matter of hours. You have to understand, I'd gone through 15 months of pure hell and Dr. Debby came along and fixed my problem in a day. It's simply amazing. I tell people there is a solution. There is someone that can find the answer and can fix you within a short time span. She gives you back your life. Without her, I don't know where I'd be - or if I'd even be. And she didn't just give my life back to me - she gave it back to my husband, my children, my grandchildren, and to all of the volunteer organizations that I can now participate in again. I'll be able to go to the Veteran's Day ceremony this November 11th solely because of the wonderful work the staff of Vision Specialists was able to do with me. It's like the ripple effect when a rock is thrown into the pond. It has affected everyone that I know and all of the organizations that I'm involved in.

People are surprised and delighted to see that I can now do all the things I used to do. Simple things like letting the dog out into the yard or going to the mailbox to get my mail.

Dr. Debby and Vision Specialists gave me back my life. Literally. My husband brought me a new car and I'm now driving! How amazing is that?! Especially when I'd been limited to just sitting on the couch for the better part of my day. It blows my mind how bad my situation was and how debilitating my life had become. I used to have to hold on to the sink just to brush my teeth. I wasn't able to do anything without assistance. When you get to that point you seriously think to yourself: *'Why am I here? I can't contribute anything to society.'* Before going to Vision Specialists, I used to just wait for the hours of the day to pass by. Now I can say I'm driving again. I'm reading to my grandchildren. I'm involved in all of the various organizations and committees I used to volunteer in. I'm able to be a positive contributor for myself and the world around me. I'm 'me' again!

What saddens me is that when I was leaving the hospital that had referred me to see Dr. Debby, there was a woman there that had traveled all the way from Alaska, and she'd been told there was nothing they could do for her. And now I really feel that Dr. Debby could've helped her just like she helped me. I just know it.

It's imperative that the work that Vision Specialists does and the knowledge they have of Vertical Heterophoria is shared with others in the medical field so that they can be trained in this special area as well. It will allow more people to have access to these much-needed services. People have to be educated not just about the problems of Vertical Heterophoria, but also about the solutions!

The Article On Vertical Heterophoria Was Describing Me

by D. F.   *Story 32*

I've been wearing glasses since I was fifteen years old. For years I didn't experience any special problems or concerns with my vision, and had adjusted to wearing glasses quite well. I didn't need to wear them full-time, mostly just for reading and studying, and was able to wear glasses for many years without a problem. As expected, by the time I reached my fifties, my vision needs started to change, and I began wearing glasses on a full-time basis.

At one point I started to notice that I would have short bouts of dizziness. This was new to me. There would be no symptoms or precursor to let me know when this dizziness would occur. I can vividly remember an incident when I was visiting one of my daughters in Philadelphia. It was about ten in the morning and I was just sitting in her living room thinking about my return flight to Detroit which was scheduled for later that afternoon. All of a sudden, the room seemed to start spinning. I wasn't moving, I hadn't attempted to stand or anything. I thought to myself: "Oh my gosh!" I stood up and I was kind of flailing around to hold onto something. Since this wasn't the first time this had happened, my daughter was aware of what was going on with me. We thought it would be best for me to get to a bedroom to lie down for a few moments, since the dizziness occurred even with my just sitting quietly. I made it into the bedroom to lie down and although I didn't feel tired at the time, my daughter did inform me that I'd fallen asleep for a short period. I wasn't able to lay for too long though, because my flight was leaving at 2:00 p.m. and I had to be at the airport at least an hour prior to that time.

The incident at my daughter's home reminded me of a previous time during a recent Easter Sunday. Towards the end of the church service I became dizzy and could not stand straight. I realized these incidents were beginning to increase in frequency and were becoming more severe. The room would seem to spin out of control and I had no idea why. Sometimes I would also get nauseous while experiencing these bouts of dizziness. As a result, I became nervous when I realized they could happen without any warning, and I began to worry about where I might be or what task I'd be performing when the dizziness would occur. I found myself having to lie down for about an hour or two in order for the symptoms to go away, or to at least subside.

One time I was lying in bed when the dizziness started, and it was accompanied by a strong feeling of nausea. I couldn't even turn my head from looking straight ahead to looking sideways without feeling quite ill. I placed a small bowl on my nightstand in case I needed to use it quickly due to the nausea. That incident lasted 1½ days. During that time I could not get out of bed for any length of time. I laid there, too dizzy and nauseous to move.

In August 2004, I noticed an article in the *Detroit Free Press* (our local paper) which featured a story about Dr. Debby and a patient with dizziness that markedly improved with a pair of glasses that had prisms in them. As I read the article and the symptoms the patient had been experiencing, I remembered thinking to myself. "Gosh—that's me! Those are the same issues I've been dealing with for some time now." The article went on to explain the work that Dr. Debby and her staff at Vision Specialists were doing with a condition called Vertical Heterophoria, and how they were able to improve vision as well as many of the other symptoms of VH with prismatic lenses. Let me tell you - I was reading that article at 7:30 in the morning, and by 8:00 that morning I was on the phone with the staff of Vision Specialists! I was able to secure an appointment with them and was excited about the possibility of not only finding out what could be causing my problems, but hopefully finding a solution to them as well.

On the day of my appointment, Dr. Debby listened to my concerns and explained to me in greater detail the work that Vision Specialists does. She began to examine me to see if I was a candidate for a pair of prism glasses. The examination was unlike any eye exam I'd ever experienced, but I didn't see it as time-consuming. Dr. Debby is very thorough in conducting the eye examination and she asks questions that at first glance don't seem to be connected with your vision concerns, but you're soon able to see the overall connection and are able to understand what it could mean for you.

I was amazed at how well the prism glasses worked for me, and just like the article I'd read earlier, not only did I receive clarity with my vision but my other symptoms were eliminated as well. I was no longer experiencing dizziness, the room did not seem to spin out of control for me, and my nausea was gone.

Shortly after receiving my new prism glasses, Dr. Debby was featured on a health segment on the six 'o clock local evening TV news. That made me think to mention it to my friends and give them the opportunity to see if Vision Specialists might be able to help them as well. Subsequently, I discovered that one of my good friends has a daughter-in-law that lives in Kentucky who had been experiencing symptoms similar to mine. She found out about Vision Specialists of Michigan, came for an examination and was also helped with prism lenses.

Vision Specialists is just across town from me - I am sure blessed that I do not have to travel from out of state to utilize their services, though I know others do travel from far and wide for help from them. I go annually to have my eyes re-examined and to have my prescription updated, and I am so glad the prism glasses were a solution for me!

I often wonder why more people are not aware of Vision Specialists and the important work that they are doing with Vertical Heterophoria, but then I remember how I, too, wasn't aware of them, and how I just happened to read that *Detroit Free Press* article on that particular day. For people who are experiencing any of the symptoms of Vertical Heterophoria, suffering through that condition can be miserable.

The scary part for me and my VH symptoms was that I just never knew what might bring on the symptoms, how long they would last, or what could be done to eliminate them. I became anxious and overwhelmed at the thought of getting through my day. For me, there were no warning signs or any indication of when my dizziness and nausea would occur. Imagine what it must be like driving, or having to work under those conditions!

Recently I returned from a trip to London, and I was elated about being able to travel, enjoy myself and move around without experiencing any dizziness or nausea. In addition, it's nice to have my vision greatly improved! I'll soon be visiting with my daughter again in Philadelphia and I'm excited and looking forward to it. It's nice not to be sick anymore, and be able to live a normal life!

To Be Symptom-Free Is Amazing!

by Joel Fallon   *Story 33*

I used to get migraines on a regular basis. Over the years I've learned to cope with them as best I could, but at times they've proven to be quite challenging. To make matters worse, once while camping, I'd taken a blow to my head and although it did not seem to be a major incident, I noticed a few months later that I started experiencing vertigo. Since the vertigo didn't begin right away, I wasn't able to make the connection between the blow to the head and the vertigo. As things began to worsen for me, I started to undergo testing to see if there had been significant damage from having hit my head while camping. The vertigo got so disabling that I started to feel like I was falling all the time and needed to regain my balance. I'd gone to different ENT's (Ear/Nose/Throat specialists) in an effort to get relief, and was told my problems had to do with having a viral infection in my inner ear and was given medication to take care of it. However, the vertigo was not alleviated. At times, I had to be off work for a short period.

A few months passed since the start of the vertigo. A couple of colleagues at work who had also been experiencing vertigo had gone to Dr. Arthur Rosner (an ENT) who thought they had a vision problem causing their vertigo, and referred them to Vision Specialists of Michigan. They excitedly told me I should see him and find out if I might need a referral there as well. After talking to a few others who were familiar with Dr. Rosner and who were recommending him to me, I thought it would make sense to at least check it out.

I saw Dr. Rosner and he confirmed that my vertigo had nothing to do with my inner ear, and that my condition was more than likely related to my eyes. This was surprising news for me because I would never have associated vertigo or being off-balance with anything having to do with my eyes. He advised me to make an appointment with Vision Specialists of Michigan. He explained the condition of Vertical Heterophoria to me. I was excited at the prospect of someone being able to not only tell me why I was experiencing vertigo, but also a possible way to make it better. I also talked with Dr. Rosner about the migraines I'd been having for years, and he told me that the Vertical Heterophoria could be causing that as well, and that it also might get better with treatment.

Initially, I didn't know what to expect. I'd reviewed some research on prism lenses and in the past the glasses were all big, bulky contraptions. I was thinking: 'What am I getting myself into?' Of course after dealing with dizziness and headache symptoms for so long and having gone to so many different specialists, by the time you're referred to a place that might be able to make a major difference in your life, you really don't care what your glasses might look like. You're more interested in whether or not they'll work for you. Little did I know that the prisms are undetectable and the glasses look like regular eyeglasses.

During my appointment at Vision Specialists of Michigan it was discovered that I did suffer from Vertical Heterophoria, and that my visual acuity was off a bit as well, and it was felt that both were contributing to my vertigo and headaches.

While I didn't experience all of the major debilitating VH symptoms over my lifetime, I had enough problems from the headaches and the vertigo that I can't imagine anyone having to suffer with VH symptoms long term. Having vertigo is one of those conditions where you find yourself unable to do the normal things you're used to doing. For me it was horrible just suffering through it for the short time that I'd had it.

I was lucky that I was referred to Dr. Rosner and was able to receive help within a few months of the start of my vertigo. That point was really brought home to me while I was being examined in the Vision Specialists office. There was a gentleman there from out of state who was a military serviceman, and he'd been dealing with his symptoms for a few years. He'd flown to Michigan to be examined by Vision Specialists. They were able to help him when no one else could, and he said he was happy to have made the trip. He told me he thought he was going to have to retire from the service due to his symptoms, but after getting his prism glasses that was no longer an issue. He'd been searching for a few years to find out what was wrong, but none of the doctors and specialists he saw were familiar with Vertical Heterophoria, so he simply wasn't able to be helped.

Since wearing my prism glasses I no longer have episodes of vertigo. The number of times I have migraines has been greatly reduced, and the headaches have lessened in their severity. I may get migraines for a few hours once a month or so, whereas before I'd been experiencing severe migraines at least twice a week and they would linger on for the majority of the day. This is a major difference for me for sure! I used to wear glasses only for reading, but now I wear my glasses all the time, and they've made a huge impact upon my daily life. When I remove them for a half-hour or so I start to experience vertigo, so I know it's the prism glasses that are making the difference. With the prism glasses I no longer have vertigo, the headaches are reduced, and my vision is improved. It has been a complete and amazing change for me!

With VH, It Takes Every Ounce of Energy Just To Get Through The Day

by Mary English   *Story 34*

My problem started fairly suddenly one evening. I'd just returned from a very active day with my family, and went to lie on the bed for a moment. My husband and son were sitting on the bed, and just the tiniest movement from them made me so nauseous that I had to go to the restroom to clear my head. From that day on, seemingly from nowhere, I would get really dizzy and my balance seemed to be off, causing me to walk awkwardly. At first, I thought I would get better and my symptoms would dissipate. But instead of getting better, they worsened. A trip to my doctors' office revealed that I had a condition called Benign Positional Vertigo.

I was referred to a Balance clinic. There I was taught some basic exercises which were designed to get my brain and my eyes back in sync with one another. The exercises didn't work for me, and I started having headaches on a daily basis. Along with the headaches I began experiencing sensitivity to light and sound, which caused my headaches to become full-blown migraines. My primary care physician referred me to a neurologist to undergo treatment for the migraines.

In the interim, I started going to different specialists for the vertigo symptoms and other issues related to being off balance. My ears were checked, but the tests were all negative. Since we weren't able to determine what was wrong, I was given medication for the migraines and a prescription to prevent seizures.

At work, I was struggling with the dizziness, nausea, and of course, the migraines. At times, I was afraid I would slide under the meeting room table and slip into a state of unconsciousness. I was beside myself. I would be in tears on a daily basis, dreading having to deal with these symptoms while trying to cope and make it through each day. I felt as if these symptoms were more than just the Benign Positional Vertigo I'd been diagnosed with.

I began to search the internet to see if there was any information as to what could possibly be wrong with me. I'd key in words like dizziness, migraines and nausea, and try to see if there were any sites that had all of these symptoms together. While doing the internet search, I stumbled upon a blog that dealt with all of these symptoms. I was so intrigued that I read the entire blog. At the end of it, there was a link to the Vision Specialists website. The questionnaire there was a pure shock to me. There they were - the symptoms I'd been having, all together in one place. And it appeared they were part of a condition: Vertical Heterophoria - it had been identified! I excitedly completed the questionnaire and submitted it, hoping I'd be able to finally understand what was going on with me.

Within two hours I received a call from Dr. Debby. I explained to her that I was preparing to drive up to one of the Mayo Clinics to have some thorough testing done, but she told me that after reviewing the on-line questionnaire that I'd submitted, she thought she might be able to provide a solution for many of my symptoms. She explained that the problem might be with my eyes, specifically the vertical alignment of my eyes. I was intrigued and hopeful and set up an appointment.

On the way to Michigan for my appointment I thought I'd be able to help with the driving. But when I tried to do so, the trees along the side of the road were casting shadows before me. The lane marking lines on the road were distracting to me, as they seemed to be coming right at me! This had never happened before. In the small area where I live, we don't have that many lane marking lines on the road and the streets are not landscaped with trees, so there are no shadows to cast. I never suspected I'd have an issue when it came to driving. I was only able to drive about 5 miles before I got horribly dizzy and my husband had to continue the trek to Michigan. I simply could not drive and was becoming physically ill trying to do so.

Dr. Debby greeted me warmly and began to explain to me the answers I'd submitted on the questionnaire and what it all meant. It was all finally coming together and making sense to me. The eye exam was the most thorough one I'd ever had with an eye doctor. She made sure that not only were my eyes comfortable when looking through a new pair of prism lenses, but that I felt physically comfortable as well, and wasn't straining or tense during the exam.

I tried on a temporary pair of the prism lenses and my migraine went away! It was unbelievable to me, but I immediately noticed that I didn't have a headache and I didn't feel any type of pressure around my head! I didn't think it was possible to feel like that simply by trying on glasses, but here I was feeling immediate relief. I couldn't wait to have my prism glasses completed so that my life could get back to normal again!

Dr. Debby advised me that as my eyes became more and more relaxed, my prescription for my prism glasses could change within the next few weeks to months, which would necessitate further exams to "fine tune" the lens prescription. I mentioned my concern about traveling from Illinois to Michigan and we agreed to try to have my regular ophthalmologist adjust the prism glasses for me. But when I did that, the ones given to me from my regular ophthalmologist simply did not work. My headaches returned, I was off balance again, and I began to have eye strain. I wound up having to go back to Dr. Debby to fine tune my prism eyeglasses. I found out that other optometrists and ophthalmologists don't follow the same methods and techniques that Vision Specialists does. Vision Specialists works with very small units of prisms and their lenses are truly customized for the needs of each individual. They conduct their exams in a very specific way to determine just the right amount of prisms for the lenses.

The lenses that Dr. Debby prescribed had a huge impact on me. I'm able to walk straight and confidently and I have my balance back. Without my prism glasses, I'd walk too close to the walls and hit a door frame when entering rooms - I don't do that when I have my prism glasses on. Also, my depth perception has improved 100%.

When I was at work prior to receiving my prism glasses, I really struggled with looking at my laptop and then across the room at the projection screen. My eyes just couldn't make the adjustment easily. My migraines were unbearable, making it even more difficult to focus or concentrate on anything at work; and that was coupled with the nausea and dizziness. I'd be extremely fatigued, and I'd get home and be exhausted. When it takes every ounce of your energy just to get through your workday, there's nothing left of you to give when you'd get home. I'd literally crash into bed and dread having to do it all again the next day.

It was necessary for me to take some time off from work due to my eye strain and other symptoms. Dr. Debby made it clear that I needed to allow my eyes to completely relax. For me, that meant taking the time to look into the distance often, but working in the environment that I was in at the time wasn't conducive for that. My time off from work allowed my eye muscles to completely relax so that Vision Specialists could work with my eyes in their natural state, allowing for the correct prescription to finally be determined. I have since been able to return to work on a part-time basis, and I am gradually getting my life back to normal.

It's strange to think of my having discovered the information for Vision Specialists by stumbling upon a blog that had a link to the on-line questionnaire that I submitted. Sometimes I think just how different my life would have been had I never come across it. Since wearing the prism glasses, I no longer need to take the medication for the migraines, as I do not experience them! For anyone that is currently experiencing migraines, you can imagine what a relief it would be to have them eliminated from your daily life!

I wish ophthalmologists and optometrists were aware of Vertical Heterophoria and the symptoms related to it. It would be a huge boon if all of the knowledge that Vision Specialists has put together on VH could be disseminated and taught so that more people could have access to these much-needed services. It would also be helpful if other health care practitioners that are not vision care providers could at least be aware of the symptoms of this condition, and make the appropriate referrals when necessary.

Most people are like me, and are not at all aware of Vertical Heterophoria and the various debilitating symptoms it could cause them to experience. I tell others that complain about headaches and dizziness to go to the website and check out the questionnaire. Dr. Debby and Vision Specialists have really helped me out a lot. I don't think I'd be where I am now if it weren't for their assistance!

Most Optometrists and Ophthalmologists Do Not Know How To Diagnose and Treat VH

by S. S.   *Story 35*

I was in the hospital about fifteen years ago for pre-term labor, and began started vertigo. I was working part-time, and was hoping that the vertigo would just be a transitional type of thing for me. I remember moving my eyes and having everything spinning and I didn't think it was normal, but I felt it was something I'd be able to deal with every now and then. So I started adjusting my life and my limitations, and over time I simply thought: *this was the way things were supposed to be for me and this is how I'm supposed to feel.* I kind of felt like something might be wrong with my eyes, so I went to see an optometrist, but she wasn't able to find anything, so I just thought, well, ok, I'll live through it.

I simply went on with life. About five years ago, I decided to go back to work full-time. Everything went well for awhile. Then about a year into having worked full-time, I began to experience headaches more often. I attributed that to the stress of getting back to working full-time, but then I also started having problems when driving. I had a 45 minute drive and found myself struggling to get to work because I felt dizzy and anxious - I'd get to work and be totally stressed out. I began thinking that maybe I should stop driving for awhile.

Shortly after noticing these symptoms, panic attacks started happening while I was driving. I'd try to calm myself down so that I could work all day, but it was overwhelming to say the least. After the day's work, I'd dread having to get behind the wheel again and experience panic attacks while I headed home. It just got to the point that I could not drive to work anymore. On top of that, I'd get home and have to be on 'mommy duty.' Soon I began to lose sleep, and the less sleep I got the worse everything was, which of course led me to be even more stressed out and anxious.

By now, I was experiencing headaches every day. For a while, family members began driving me to work and picking me up, but finally they suggested I go get checked out to see what exactly was causing these symptoms and what could be done about them. My doctor advised me to take a leave from work, which was a huge financial and emotional struggle for me. I underwent a series of tests, and was referred to an ENT (Ear/Nose/Throat) specialist and a neurologist. An MRI was ordered, and other tests and treatment for my migraines were scheduled. It was thought that the vertigo and dizziness were related to the migraines, so that was the main focus. I had been dealing with the vertigo symptoms for many years already at this point, but this type of dizziness felt different than what I'd grown used to. I had been given new medications to take, but I wound up having to stop those medications because I felt it was making my dizziness worse. It may have helped with the headaches, but the dizziness was causing a lot of stress all of the time.

I wanted to return to work on a part-time basis but I still had problems driving. I was hoping that working just part-time would allow me more time to rest and prepare for the day. It was still exhausting, but I just kept plugging along.

As time went on, I began to compensate for the symptoms I was experiencing. I did whatever I could when I could, but nothing beyond that. I was able to take my kids back and forth to school, but only because it was a short distance. If I didn't feel like I could drive safely to the store, I just didn't go. Then I noticed that I would have to sleep before going to pick my kids up from school, just to give my eyes a rest before having to do that type of task. I went through times when I'd stay up all night just to get something done, but then that would throw me off for about a month, with me trying to sleep during the day, and being too tired to accomplish much of anything.

There would be times when I'd be sitting at a red light and my head would be spinning, and just to move my eyes slightly was painful. It was very scary and frustrating for me because I just didn't know what was wrong.

Once, I was driving back with my kids from a basketball camp and I could not get us home. I was having so much dizziness that it led to anxiety, and I had to call a family member to come out and get us. I had to be rescued like this on more than one occasion. I just did not feel safe when driving and I'd pull over and explain to my kids that mommy was fine but I just didn't feel right behind the wheel.

As my symptoms intensified, I started thinking that perhaps I had Multiple Sclerosis or Lou Gehrig's disease or some other serious ailment. You worry and hope that it's nothing major, and hope a few vitamins can help. Yet still I knew that something wasn't right. I went back to the doctor many times but usually it was during the times I'd been experiencing massive anxiety. I would get so much pressure behind my eyes, and once even had a broken blood vessel on one of my eyes. The doctors were focusing on those symptoms and all the while I kept thinking: *If I could just find the right ophthalmologist.* The MRI's were coming back fine, but still I was experiencing all of these symptoms.

I was beginning to realize the ridiculous lengths I was going through to just get things done on a daily basis now, and thought about how much all of this was affecting family members who were trying to help support me by coming to my aid whenever I called on them. I just didn't have the get-up-and-go in life that I used to have. I was always tired. I kept telling myself that I was not a lazy person, I just couldn't deal with what I had to deal with.

There were times during the winter and during early morning hours when everything was worse. Those circular ramps on the freeway caused me so much anxiety that I looked for and found a different route to work. All of these symptoms were completely affecting my life, while all the time I was trying to convince myself that everything was fine just the way it was, that everyone else must be feeling like this, too.

My mom was always my biggest supporter and she would say things like: *'This isn't you. What's wrong?'* And she tried to help me as much as she could by explaining to me that the coping mechanisms I had developed were not normal. One of the best things my mom was able to do for me was to refer me to Dr. Debby. My mom had this hair-dresser she was going to, and she'd started to discuss with her the symptoms I was experiencing. The hairdresser excitedly told my mom about Dr. Debby and Vision Specialists and how they were able to make some remarkable changes for others like me. My mom came to me and said: *'I've got a number you've got to call. My friend has a sister-in-law that was going through what you seem to be experiencing, and this doctor was able to help her and it changed her life. I bet it could change your life too!'*

I'll never forget the day I looked up Vision Specialists on-line. I went on the website and read the information and I immediately started to cry. Up to that point, I had started thinking I was just crazy. To see these symptoms (all of which I had) and to have them all listed in one place to me was like seeing a miracle. I remember thinking: *"Wow, this sounds exactly like me!"* I was just starting to have problems with going to the mall, and going into stores like Target or Kohl's and I would feel anxious and weird and I would think: *"This doesn't make sense. I used to love shopping at those stores."* I'd gotten to the point where I felt funny going to concerts and baseball games - things I'd loved doing in the past, but that now caused so much stress and anxiousness for me.

So when I read the website, I said: *"Finally an explanation! This is me and someone knows what's happening."* So I took the survey right away and within minutes I got a call from Dr. Debby. At first I thought it was a member of her staff, but it was her in person on the phone. She was very receptive to the information I shared with her, and she encouraged me to speak with her staff to arrange an appointment as soon as possible. Even then it was a month before I could get an appointment, but I felt so excited about the possibility of feeling even the slightest relief that I couldn't wait for that time to meet with her. I read some of the results from other patients on the website, but I didn't think I was as sick as they were, so I honestly didn't think the prism glasses would make a major difference for me, but I thought: *"As long as I feel comfortable behind the wheel again, I'll be happy. "*

For my first appointment, I went without expecting a whole lot initially, and after the exam I was given the trial glasses with the prism. To my surprise, all of my neck and back tension was immediately released! Everything looked clearer and it was so amazing to me, that I sat there overwhelmed. I was thinking: *"Oh my God. "* The first thing I did was to call my mom to thank her for recommending Vision Specialists, and then I called my husband. I told him how much relief I had gotten from just this first appointment. The second thing I noticed (besides the relief of the neck and back pain) was that I was able to get in my car and sit comfortably with my back against the seat. I hadn't been able to do that in a long time, as I was always tense and sat close to the steering wheel, but now I was fully relaxed.

Things weren't perfect in the beginning. I had an adjustment period to go through, as I had not worn glasses at all before. It took a few more eye exams to tweak my prescription, but now my glasses are wonderful - I no longer have the dizziness or the vertigo or the feelings of being overwhelmed or anxious anymore. All that had been due to my eyes straining and the rest of my body trying to compensate for that.

Prior to getting the prism glasses, just looking at the computer screen or making the movement of looking down and then looking back up would cause dizziness for me. The muscles in my eyes were struggling against each other and not feeling relaxed. My eye muscles would feel so tight it felt like suction cups were pulling on my eyeballs - that's the best way I can describe how it felt physically.

It's kind of sad, but I now remember having seen a clip about Vision Specialists a few years before my mom had recommended them to me. But the optometrists I'd been going to weren't able to diagnose what was wrong or prescribe any type of relief for me, and I thought, *'Been there, done that – it must not be my eyes.'* My skepticism kept me from checking it out then. I had no idea that most optometrist and ophthalmologist don't know about VH.

I'm so glad my mom talked with her hairdresser about my symptoms, because if she hadn't, I would never have gone to Vision Specialists and Dr. Debby. My family has definitely witnessed a change in me, as they no longer have to come to my rescue or take me to and from work. My sister came to my home and saw a difference just in the way I was able to take care of things after getting the prism glasses. My husband is able to be relieved of having to do so much to help me compensate. And it's so nice to now feel comfortable behind the wheel. I like to drive now and am no longer afraid to do so.

It's believed that I've had this condition since birth, and when you're younger, your brain and your body are able to compensate in areas that are lacking, but as we age, our bodies become weary from years of having over-worked its muscles, and you may begin to experience these symptoms. Sometimes you may experience many of the symptoms all at once, and for others it may be just a few symptoms that occur gradually.

The staff at Vision Specialists is very thorough during the exams. They pay attention to detail and they're truly passionate and care about each of their patients.

What I thought was really neat was when, during the exam, Dr. Debby instructed me not to strain when reading the letters, but to only read what was comfortable. In past eye exams I would strain to see the smallest line possible, but that's really not the right thing to do because the prescription is then based on our eyes having to strain, and then we wonder why our prescription glasses don't seem effective!

I used to drive white-knuckled, with my head close to the steering wheel, all tense, afraid of the lights at night. I used to have headaches, vertigo, nausea, fear of heights and wasn't able to drive. I no longer feel that way. Now that I'm feeling better, I look back and realize how crappy I was feeling before, and how hard it was to maintain some semblance of normalcy (even with utilizing the help of my family members). It's just amazing how much better things are now. The message I'd like to share with the wonderful staff at Vision Specialists is: Thank you. You have all been wonderful in helping me to get a new lease on life. I am very grateful for having found out about Vision Specialists and Dr. Debby in particular. My mom said it would change my life, and it truly has!

I Can Feel The Ground!

By Ana Piqueras   *Story 36*

'I can feel the ground,' may appear to be a strange thing for an ordinary person to exclaim, but the symptoms I'd been experiencing for the previous thirteen years did not allow me to have that normal, expected sensation. Instead, I experienced a type of floating, disconnected sensation. It is hard to put into words really - although I was walking, I physically could not feel the ground beneath me. Believe me, if you're walking but not able to actually feel your very foundation underfoot, it doesn't leave you confident enough to continue to place one foot in front of the other.

Unfortunately, having that sense of unbalance was the least of my worries. I had a myriad of symptoms plaguing my body for over a decade which included headaches, dizziness, double-vision, anxiety in crowded places, and a feeling of disconnectedness while walking even short distances.

It's been said that one finds ways to cope with difficult situations as they arise in our lives, and for me, I coped with the sensation of not being able to 'feel the ground' by wearing ankle weights. At least they gave me a truer sense of balance and some stability. But the weights were just a coping mechanism. The real reason I was experiencing what I was feeling, and how to confront those issues, still needed to be addressed.

Having been healthy for the majority of my life, and now having health issues that became more debilitating as time wore on without being able to define why I was suddenly experiencing them was very challenging for me.

Thus began the arduous process of going to different health care professionals in various fields of practice in an effort to determine first of all, what was causing my symptoms, and secondly, to develop a plan to treat them. I saw numerous professionals, from doctors that treat allergies to chiropractors and ENT specialists. I'd even undergone surgeries that I'd been told would alleviate symptoms, but the intended results were either temporary at most, or non-existent altogether.

As you can imagine, I was given a myriad of prescriptions over the years to combat my symptoms, and it seems I was prone to experiencing whatever side-effects they caused.

At one point, it was painful to even slightly move my head or neck. I was no longer able to attend church, go to the mall, or even grocery shop alone. My husband was my greatest support system, He steadied me when walking and assisted me in lots of other areas over the years.

One day my daughter, while reading a medical journal, ran across information about the work that Dr. Debby of Vision Specialists does with patients that were experiencing many of the symptoms that I had. My daughter shared that information with me, and I was able to take the on-line survey. Shortly thereafter, I was able to speak directly with Dr. Debby, who advised me that I might be a perfect candidate for a pair of the prism glasses. After having tried so many different techniques, surgeries, and various prescriptions, I was willing to try anything that could give me even the slightest possibility of relief. I had traveled from my home in Carey, North Carolina before to various specialists and clinics, so I said to my husband: "Let's go to Michigan!"

Vision Specialists' entire staff works really well with their patients from the moment you walk through the door. They spend the kind of individual time with you that allows them to really understand what you are experiencing. Dr. Debby has a wonderful group of people on her staff, and she sincerely cares about helping people.

Upon seeing Dr. Debby, I was advised in order to receive the maximum benefit from the prism glasses, I would have to be weaned off of the medications I was taking (in conjunction with my other doctors who were prescribing these medicines). I was more than happy to do so, and I looked forward to not having to take so many different medications all of the time.

Before getting the prism glasses I couldn't do any traveling, or do much of anything. But now I can go anywhere, and I can do what I like. Last year, I was able to visit Yellowstone Park! I'm back to going to church and doing my volunteer work, and I've even gone walking on the beach for two hours! I wasn't able to do any of those things before getting my prism glasses from Vision Specialists. A very big portion of my life has been given back to me. I feel like a different person! *I'm completely off of all of the medications I'd been taking and I feel great!* My family is really happy with my prism glasses, and with the fact that I didn't have to have additional surgeries or be given more medications.

I'll never forget the moment I first realized the difference the prism glasses were making for me. *I could feel the ground!* I have to tell you, I actually started to run around in the house. My husband was elated! He asked me what I was doing and I said: I can feel the ground! You see, with some treatments, it's a gradual process before you notice that you're feeling better. But with prism glasses, it was like, 'Boom!' And it was really amazing for me! It was a completely different feeling. I was able to get rid of the ankle weights and still feel grounded and connected.

For people who have even a few of the symptoms that I had, I tell them all about Vision Specialists and the work that Dr. Debby and her staff is doing. It's important that others have this information easily available to them, so they do not have to experience years of futile searching for answers or be subjected to the frustration of not knowing what is going on with them. Most people just assume they have to live with the dizziness and headaches, when in reality, there's a possibility that they don't.

After going to so many doctors and their not being able to define what was happening with me, I thought I was dying. And then I became afraid and didn't want to be alone, not sure what might happen to me. Eventually I began to wonder if it was just all in my head - I wondered if I was going crazy or just losing my mind. But when I really focused on what I was experiencing, I realized it was not in my head.

I also want people to know that sometimes working with the prism lenses can take some time. While you will probably notice an immediate difference with many of your symptoms, you most likely will need to have the prescription modified to gain the maximum benefit. When I got my first pair of prism glasses, many of my symptoms improved but I was still experiencing some dizziness. Dr. Debby made sure to find out which of my symptoms persisted, and then tweaked the prescription to reduce those symptoms.

Vision Specialists really changed my life. Were it not for my daughter, who's a physician, reading that medical journal, I would not have known about Vision Specialists at all, and I would still be a mess. My good days now vastly outnumber my bad days. I feel so fortunate.

Part Five

Miscellaneous Stories

I Was Labeled A Stubborn Young Lad Who Refused To Read

by Jan Homan

Initially, I had not been aware that I was experiencing vision problems, except what I considered normal issues which generally leads one to have your eyes checked. I was in my thirties before I started wearing glasses. I started off by getting reading glasses that assisted me to read the *New York Times*, which I read regularly. As the years wore on though, my reading glasses were no longer working as well, and when having my eyes checked, I was diagnosed with astigmatism and my eyeglasses were changed to a bifocal lens.

I grew up in Europe, and was just entering school age when World War II began. Looking back over the years, I remember being labeled as a stubborn young lad who refused to read. Even though I tried really hard to learn my school subjects, I was an unsuccessful student. My parents disciplined me in an effort to get me to conform, but to no avail. I wound up flunking out of all of the different schools my parents enrolled me in. I come from a very strict, traditional, religious family and to add to my angst, I'd also been born left-handed. While that's not an issue for people today, for those of us born 75 years ago it was considered a bad omen to be left-handed, and parents used different techniques to encourage their children to use their right hand predominantly. As a young boy, this caused even more stress and confusion for me. During my childhood, my parents, my teachers and our ministry made it clear to me that there was something wrong with me. I felt embarrassed in the fact that I seemed to be a grave disappointment to everyone - especially my parents.

Through much study and discipline I gradually and painstakingly taught myself how to read, but I wasn't able to accomplish that until my later years.

With all of the struggles I experienced with my family life and environment, I struck out on my own at an early age and came to the United States. I settled down, married and began a family life. When one of my children was in the 3rd grade, a teacher called us in to discuss his progress. At that time we were told our son was dyslexic. This was many years ago, and dyslexia was a fairly new concept. We were advised that one of the major challenges with dyslexia was the problems it caused with reading and deciphering letters and numbers. As this teacher was explaining all of this to us, I began to think: 'That's exactly what it was like for me when I was my son's age!' During my own youth dyslexia was even less known.

When having my son tested, I also took the initiative to have myself tested, and was also diagnosed with being dyslexic. It was a revelation! I was finally able to understand why I'd struggled so much in my youth with my studies. I now knew why I couldn't understand my subjects, and I realized that I wasn't lazy or incompetent. I had a condition that had not been known at the time and therefore had not been addressed. It did not change my past, but it certainly allowed me to make peace with it and with myself. I no longer had to wonder or worry what was wrong with me, or to blame myself for not being able to do all of the things I'd struggled with for so long.

One day, my wife happened upon a TV program that featured Dr. Debby and Vertical Heterophoria. She noted that the symptoms which Dr. Debby was describing matched many of the concerns we'd experienced with our daughter Katrina over the years. She excitedly called Katrina and advised her that the next time she visited with us she should make an appointment at Vision Specialist of Michigan.

After Katrina experienced significant improvement with her prism glasses, she excitedly talked with me about also having my eyes checked. She advised me that she'd spoken with Dr. Debby about my own reading problems and that I might have a misalignment of the eyes, too. She suggested I escort her to her next appointment and arrange to have an eye exam as well.

When I finally acquiesced, I was more than half-convinced from what my daughter had told me already, so I wasn't skeptical or anything. I was able to complete the in-depth eye exam and to speak at length with Dr. Debby, who explained in great detail (and in terms that I could easily understand) why prism lenses work and her own personal research that she'd been conducting. I felt really comfortable about the visit, and the information made sense to me.

As part of the exam, you walk along the corridor prior to receiving the prism lens and then again after, and we were able to note a marked difference between the two. Without the prisms I had a definite lean in my gait that I had not been aware of previously.

The prism lenses not only helped with my vision, but it also helped with my balance and with walking. I used to walk in a slight arc-shape formation. The prism glasses have corrected that for me. Now when I walk my dog in my neighborhood, I walk in a straight line.

Due to my own history and experience with society not knowing about Vertical Heterophoria (or even dyslexia) during my youth,

239

one of my goals is to get this information out to educators and others who work with children. Had we had this important knowledge then, it would have helped me significantly in all areas of my life. Not just with my education, but with my chosen career (which was Marketing), and certainly with my own son and his reading difficulties. If there's any way possible to get children examined earlier, we might be able to determine if a problem with their visual acuity or visual alignment is playing a key role in what seems to be a learning disability. If it can be determined that they have VH and are candidates for prism glasses, we can enhance the quality of their lives immensely. For students who are struggling with the symptoms of VH, it wreaks havoc on their self-confidence, they're not as out-going or out-spoken, and they hesitate to volunteer in class or within group settings. Once we begin to educate people about VH and start screening for it and treating it, we may find out many children who we've labeled with the terms 'learning / reading disabled' or 'dyslexic' are not disabled or dyslexic at all.

Just in my family alone, three members have been helped significantly and tremendously with prism glasses - my wife, my daughter and myself. My goal is to also have my son tested.

Prior to getting my prism glasses, when I drove for long periods, I noticed that I would become fatigued and the letters on the road signs would appear to be on top of one another, resulting in the road signs looking garbled. I could solve the problem by closing one of my eyes, but of course that not only takes away my depth perception, it simply is not a solution when driving. With my prism glasses, fatigue no longer occurs with me unless I've just stayed up too late and am really physically tired overall.

I must admit that I had some anger and resentment as I wondered why I had to wait so long to be diagnosed and treated for VH. I was angry that this information wasn't readily available when I was young. Sometimes you can't help but feel a tinge of bitter resentment over the years that were spent trying to figure this thing out. It kept me from getting any formal education, which is something I surely would've pursued. That's not to say I wasn't able to make a comfortable life for myself, but there were plenty of opportunities that I simply wasn't able to take advantage of due to my VH symptoms. In retrospect, I have to understand that I grew up during a time when none of the things we now know today about VH were available to any of us back then. I realize there's no one to blame, and I'm very grateful for the help that I've been able to receive, even at this late stage of my life (I am in my 70's). With my prism glasses I am seeing well, I am able to read my *New York Times* (which I love doing), I am walking better and I am much more confident than I've ever been.

If Only All Eye Doctors Knew About This

by Katrina H.   *Story 38*

My story began when I started to have major problems driving on the highway. I found that my eyes would get really tired, particularly whenever I had to shift my focus from looking at the dashboard area back to looking at the road. I would have this funny feeling that my eyesight wasn't working right. That was very disconcerting, especially when driving on the highway, which has its own obstacles to contend with (like the fast pace of the traffic and being really aware of the other drivers around you) and I would become very anxious about it. More and more I began to avoid driving alone on the highway; and even when I'd have a passenger, I would still be uncomfortable.

In order to be able to drive long distances, I had to be feeling really good. By that I mean I had to plan for it. I had to be well-rested, being sure not to involve myself in any activity or event that would tire me out beforehand. I found it really interesting that other people could work all day, and then get in their cars and drive and seem to be quite alright with it, because that simply was not the case with me.

When I was in college I began to wear reading glasses. I was fine with that because I felt that's a period in your life when you're spending the bulk of your time reading and being on the computer. I had glasses with prisms back then, but the prisms were too strong. Unlike Dr. Debby at Vision Specialists, my eye doctor from years ago did not work with the small increments of prism. My glasses did not work for me at all because they hurt my eyes, and as a result it was too challenging for me to wear them.

At some point in my early twenties, I began tilting my head so that I could see things evenly and more precisely. I had no idea that my vision was causing the head tilt and that my vision needed to be aligned.

I moved away from Michigan, but my parents still lived there. One day my mom happened to catch some news program that was showcasing the work that was being performed on VH by Dr. Debby at Vision Specialists. She noticed that Dr. Debby was describing many of the symptoms that I'd been experiencing over the years. My mom called to tell me all about it, and she seemed really enthused. She encouraged me to make an appointment with Vision Specialists during my next planned visit home.

The best part of my initial eye-exam (apart from getting a prism prescription that was just right for me) was when I began to explain to Dr. Debby what it felt like dealing with all of my symptoms. She was so familiar with them that she was able to finish my sentences, or give an apt description of what it was I was trying to say but wasn't able to (because I was having a hard time finding the right words). I found myself saying: "That's *exactly* what I'm talking about!" It was a relief to finally find an optometrist that not only listened to what I had to say, but that really understood how I felt. The questions that she asked me during the exam really got to the heart of the issues that I was having, and it was clear to me that she really would be able to help me with my eyes. I felt confident that a difference could be made for me.

During the eye exam, I noticed that Dr. Debby always ended her instructions with the words 'without effort'. I thought that was interesting, and it made total sense to me. Under normal conditions I shouldn't have to strain and struggle to see - I should be relaxed and focused on what I'm seeing. The eye exam should be under the same conditions. Dr. Debby said this method gives her the most accurate information for the lens prescription.

When I got my prism glasses, the improvement in some of my symptoms was immediately noticeable. Since I no longer had to tilt my head to see clearly, my neck pain was diminished and the shoulder pain I'd been experiencing daily was dramatically reduced (the shoulder pain won't go away completely though because I'd injured it earlier in life).

I can now see clearly and read things in the distance and it feels great! I am comfortable and confident in what I can do with my eyes now. I no longer have the anxiousness or stress when driving anymore.

Upon returning home to Connecticut, one of my goals was to try to find an eye doctor in my area that does the type of work that Vision Specialists does, but I haven't been able to find any facilities that are even familiar with the small units of prisms she prescribes. I've been told they simply don't use prisms that small. It's hard for me to get them to understand that while it may seem 'small' by traditional standards, it is just the right amount for the prescription that I need – the one that makes such a huge difference for me, my eyes and my symptoms. I just keep thinking: *'If only all eye-doctors knew about this.'* I'm fortunate that my parents still live in Michigan, because when I visit them I also make my eye appointment with Vision Specialists to update my prescription, as my eyes and my lens prescriptions (including the prism) do change over the years.

Our eyes are used all the time and are connected to many of our body's other systems. If your eyes hurt, sometimes it can cause headaches, which can bring on a sense of dizziness or anxiety, which can in turn cause one to feel nauseous. It's important for people to understand that the body is really one unit and it's all connected to itself.

Getting the word out on VH is challenging for one person or one clinic to do, and it's important that people have the opportunity to get to know about this condition. For instance, can you imagine what an impact it would make for people who are educators, or who work on a daily basis with kids? They'd be able to notice when students are having difficulty copying from the board; or notice when they're tilting their heads; or really be in tune to hear when they're complaining about the glasses they wear - not because they don't want to wear them, but because they cause dizziness or headaches or other issues. They can observe students who are having problems reading or concentrating, and discover it's because they're not seeing things clearly; or the glasses they currently have just may not be right for them.

It's a good thing my mom happened to catch Dr. Debby on that morning news show, because not only did I benefit from their services, but my parents now have prism glasses that have had a positive impact on them as well!

You Just Don't Realize How Your Vision Is Affecting You Until The Prism Glasses Make You Better!

by Tim Jundt   *Story 39*

In the beginning, I really wasn't aware of having any unique problems in relation to my vision. I'd compensated for my shortcomings my entire life without even knowing that I was adapting to a little known condition called Vertical Heterophoria (VH). Quite honestly it appears that this condition simply is not an area of basic study in the health care field and for the most part is unheard of.

All during my school years I did really well academically, but for the entire time it was quite a struggle. In college, I spent over twice the time in my studies than many of my friends, as I found I had to really focus on comprehending what I read, and in many instances, I relegated myself to simply memorizing everything. Spelling and reading were also difficult, as I had to reread pages over and over in my attempt to grasp the information.

I was never able to do well in any sport that required hand-eye coordination, such as baseball, basketball or video games with my grand-children, and I would become frustrated with my poor performance in those activities. Even when I gave it my all and focused my attention on these activities, I was still unable to improve.

I was told I had ADD. (Attention Deficit Disorder) While I personally did not think that was the case, I did notice when in group settings and listening to speakers, my attention would go astray. I would lose interest in the speaker, and would begin to do other things to occupy myself.

Years passed with my having adapted to various symptoms such as tilting my head, getting headaches, becoming fatigued when reading, having to reread pages over and over in order to comprehend them, and motion sickness.

Over the recent years, my family began to research holistic ways to achieve better health. One of the chiropractors we began working with asked me to close my eyes and complete a type of adjustment that we normally do while there. Afterwards I was asked to do the same regimen, but this time with my eyes opened. It was noted that with my eyes closed I passed most of the regimented tasks, but with my eyes opened I did not. This doctor advised me that the tests indicated there might be problems with my eyes and my vision, and referred me to Vision Specialists of Michigan.

I wasn't sure what to expect during my exam at Vision Specialists. I wasn't skeptical, but I hadn't bought in to the entire concept of it, either. That is, until the optometrist had me conduct a horizontal test. She had me look through the phoropter (the machine with all the knobs and dials that the eye doctor places in front of your face to figure out your lens prescription) and asked me to let her know when two objects became even with each other. When I did, she moved away the phoropter and had me look at the results. I was astonished at how far off they actually were, almost by 7 inches! She then explained to me how Vertical Heterophoria is a condition that involves the misalignment of the eyes, and it all made sense to me.

I was given prism test glasses to wear during my first office visit and was instructed to sit in the waiting area for a few moments to allow me to adjust to them. The immediate changes I felt were indescribable. Even now, when talking about it, that same emotion washes over me. After years of not having had that connection with my vision, there's just no way to describe it.

I noticed many immediate changes. I was able to pay attention to speakers and participate within group settings without any difficulty at all. My comprehension in reading was dramatically increased. I was no longer tilting my head. I did not have to reread pages in order to grasp the information. I did not become fatigued when reading after a short while, and in fact am able to read for longer periods of time without getting headaches.

A success story about my prism glasses I'd like to share involves an activity that occurred while on a family vacation. I was playing a video game called Mario-Cart with my grandsons and sons-in-laws, which requires one to be adept at hand-eye coordination. As you can imagine, the testosterone levels were high and while the competition was friendly, it was no secret that we all wanted to end as champions. I was able to win at that particular game. It felt fantastic! Well, the next day, they wanted to play the game again, and because we were doing some water-sports earlier in the day, I'd been wearing my contacts (but not my prism glasses). I didn't think much of it and we began to play the game again. I did terrible! I was losing. I was not having fun with the game and I couldn't understand how my performance could have changed so drastically from the night before. I became frustrated and called it quits after a short while. I retired early for the night and while lying in bed, I kept wondering what was different from the previous day. Then it dawned on me - I'd been playing the game today without my prism glasses! Needless to say, the next day when the challenge for the game was on, I wore my prism glasses and believe it or not—I won! I wasn't the top winner, but I came in second. I tell you, there was nothing like that feeling of achievement and enjoying activities with my family while on vacation.

In another story I'd like to share, there's a group of guys that I get together with once in awhile to play basketball. On this day we were playing pool basketball. Normally I don't do too well, and I'm one of the guys that is chosen last for teams, but we're all friends and we just play for fun, so it's no big deal. Well this time, I was able to see clearly and my hand-eye coordination was right on target, I made every basket I shot, and again I won! The guys were all asking what I did differently. It was a great feeling, and the change was due to the prism glasses I was now wearing.

Lastly, I wanted to share a story that seemed so surreal for me. I was opening a cabinet, and a cup and saucer started to tumble out inadvertently. Although I was startled, I was able to catch both of them separately with one hand! It sounds a bit corny, but *I felt like a super-hero!* My reactions were like Spider-man and I thought: 'In the past, I never would have been able to do that.' It was just really cool.

The information about VH is not yet widespread, and I certainly would like to help in getting this information out to others. I was fortunate that in my case, my doctor was made aware of the work Vision Specialists does via a network of holistic practitioners and he was able to refer me to them.

Everything I do, from hand-eye coordination to mental activities - it is all definitely easier since I've received my prism glasses. Now when reading, I'm able to do so without becoming distracted or having to reread sentences, and my comprehension is complete. I no longer have a difficult time when reading and I no longer dread doing so. My motion sickness has not been completely eliminated, but it is not nearly as bad as it had been before. You really don't realize how bad your vision is until you put the correct set of glasses on for the first time and now all of sudden you can see. You can see the details of the clouds, the nuances of colors and other things which were not quite as clear or in focus to you before. My whole body now feels better, as it no longer needs to fight against itself to achieve proper eye alignment. I'm much more comfortable in my environment and much more confident with the tasks that I'm performing. I must sincerely say with my prism glasses, *life is easier!*

I Never Thought My Symptoms Had Anything To Do With My Eyes

by R. E. U.   *Story 40*

As I look back in my life, I realize that many of the symptoms that I'd been experiencing actually started quite a long time ago, prior to my high school years. Symptoms such as feeling pressure behind my eyes that left my muscles across my forehead feeling tense and taut. I had a general feeling of motion sickness that was always with me even when I wasn't in cars or traveling. I also began having anxiety attacks.

Later, driving on the freeway was a problem for me, as well as trouble with escalators. I'd have to be really cautious getting on and off of both of them, and doing so would trigger a rush of anxiety for me. Being on an escalator for just a few moments would cause me to feel as if I would fall backwards. I would get dizzy and anxious and I never knew why.

Soon, I was afraid to go to stores in the mall because of my anxiety attacks. I used to love going to the mall! I had no idea what was going on with me and I gradually began to isolate myself and withdrew from society more and more.

As my symptoms became worse and began intruding on my daily life, I sought answers. I went to a therapist for awhile who prescribed some medications to ease some of my symptoms, but the major problem I was having with my eyes (which seem to be causing many of the other issues) did not go away.

I found out about Vision Specialists from my sister. Her daughter had been experiencing symptoms similar to what had been plaguing me for years. My sister excitedly explained to me that the entire time she'd been completing Vision Specialists' on-line survey for her daughter, the more she realized how I had many of these same symptoms. She remembered what life was like for me when we were growing up, and she was convinced that Vision Specialists may be able to help me as well. She'd explained how her daughter had experienced marked improvement with a pair of the prism glasses, and encouraged me to call for an appointment. I told her I'd give them a try, but I never thought any of these symptoms would have anything to do with my eyes at all.

After reviewing the information on the Vision Specialists' website, I began to wonder if it could be possible to have some of my symptoms alleviated. I was anxious to go for my first appointment because I thought it would be really cool to find out what was wrong overall, and to see if there was really something that could be done about it. I wasn't really expecting much, because I still didn't understand what Vertical Heterophoria was, and I wasn't confident as to what could be done for me personally. I did not want to get my hopes up, but after I met with Dr. Debby, who confirmed I had the misalignment of the eyes, it was a great relief for me. I now had a name for what was going on and I began to look forward to getting better.

Once I received my pair of prism glasses my entire life changed! Within the first week I was able to notice the anxiety (that had been a mainstay with me when driving) was no longer an issue. I was able to merge onto the freeway successfully and without panicking or having anxiety. Before when driving, if I were in the middle lane with cars on both sides of me, I'd always felt like I was actually going backwards which would cause the anxiety attacks. Just imagine how you would feel if you're driving along the freeway feeling as if you're going backwards! It was sheer joy being able to drive normally

Being able to finally be in control in many other areas of my life was also a boost for my self-esteem. I can remember once, prior to getting my prism glasses, I'd mentally psyched myself up to go to the mall. At the mall, I walked over into the center area to begin my trek down the corridor, but I immediately began to have an anxiety attack and I had to leave. I felt so bad and confused. With my prism glasses, I can now just jump into the car, go to the mall, do everything that I need to do and actually enjoy that time without experiencing anxiety or feeling as if I won't be able to complete my shopping. I no longer have to shy away from everyday tasks, and that is a major improvement in my life. Even my motion sickness is gone.

Seeing major improvements with the prism glasses is great, but realizing the many little improvements is awesome as well. My social life has improved because I no longer feel as if I have to shield myself from society. I am more confident and independent. I don't worry about anxiety attacks and the motion sickness is completely gone. In fact for me, the motion sickness or experiencing problems on escalators are now indicators that it's time to have my lenses updated. When I begin to experience either of those, I know it's time to make a new eye appointment!

For me, it was my sister, while trying to find a solution for the problems her daughter was having, who recognized that I had similar symptoms and recommended me to Vision Specialists. Were it not for that, I fear that I would still be experiencing all of the symptoms I had, which were worsening over the years. If you or someone you know is experiencing problems that may or may not seem to be connected with your vision or your eyes, it may be helpful to review the information at the Vision Specialist website, or speak with your optometrist or health care professional to see if they're familiar with Vertical Heterophoria. Like me, you may be a candidate for a pair of prism glasses and are simply unaware of it. Wouldn't it be worth it to find out? It certainly has been worth it for me!

APPENDIX A

How To Score The Adult VHSQ

The Adult Vertical Heterophoria Symptom Questionnaire (VHSQ) has been designed to detect those patients 18 years old and older whose headache, dizziness, anxiety or neck ache might be due to a visually mediated cause (usually Vertical Heterophoria). Feel free to make a copy of the questionnaire and use it yourself, or give it to a friend or loved one you suspect might have VH. Scoring is performed by summing the values given to <u>Questions 1 – 25 only</u> as follows:

Always = 3

Frequently = 2

Occasionally = 1

Never = 0

If the score is $\geq$ 15, consultation with a Neurovisual optometrist is recommended.

Vertical Heterophoria Symptom Questionnaire (VHSQ)

for those 18 years old and older

Vision Specialists of Michigan

2550 S. Telegraph Road, Suite 100   Bloomfield Hills, Michigan 48302   (248) 258-9000
www.VSofM.com   Fax (248) 499-6372

Name: _____   Email: _____   Date: _____

Best phone number: _____   Back-up phone number: _____

Directions: For each of the following questions, please check the answer that best describes your situation. If you wear glasses or contact lenses, answer the questions assuming that you are wearing them. Please answer every question.

Always = Everyday
Frequently = At least 1 time / week
Occasionally = Less than 1 time / week
Never = Never

	ALWAYS	FREQUENTLY	OCCASIONALLY	NEVER
1. Do you have headaches and / or facial pain?				

2. Do you have pain in your eyes with eye movement?

3. Do you experience neck or shoulder discomfort?

4. Do you have dizziness and / or lightheadedness?

5. Do you experience dizziness, light-headedness, or nausea while performing close-up activities (i.e. - computer work, reading, writing)?

6. Do you experience dizziness, light-headedness, or nausea while performing far-distance activities (i.e. - driving, television, movies)?

7. Do you experience dizziness, light-headedness, or nausea when bending down and standing back up, or when getting up quickly from a seated position?

8. Do you feel unsteady with walking, or drift to one side while walking?

9. Do you feel overwhelmed or anxious while walking in a large department store (i.e. – Target, Wal-Mart, Meijer)?

10. Do you feel overwhelmed or anxious when in a crowd?

11. Does riding in a car make you feel dizzy or uncomfortable?

	ALWAYS	FREQUENTLY	OCCASIONALLY	NEVER
12. Do you experience anxiety or nervousness because of your dizziness?				
13. Do you ever find yourself with your head tilted to one side?				
14. Do you experience poor depth perception or have difficulty estimating distances accurately?				
15. Do you experience double / overlapping / shadowed vision at far distances?				
16. Do you experience double / overlapping / shadowed vision at near distances?				
17. Do you experience glare or have sensitivity to bright lights?				
18. Do you close or cover one eye with near or far tasks?				
19. Do you skip lines or lose your place while reading (do you use your finger or a ruler or other guides to maintain your position on the page)?				
20. Do you tire easily with close-up tasks (computer work, reading, writing)?				
21. Do you experience blurred vision with far-distance activities (i.e. - driving, television, movies, chalkboard at school)?				

			YES	NO
			YES	NO

22. Do you experience blurred vision with close-up activities (i.e. - computer work, reading, writing)?

23. Do you blink to "clear up" distant objects after working at a desk or working with close-up activities (i.e. - computer work, reading, writing)?

24. Do you experience words running together with reading?

25. Do you experience difficulty with reading or reading comprehension?

26. Have you ever had difficulty adjusting to or being fit with previous pairs of glasses?

27. Do any other family members have problems similar to yours?

28. If you have motion sickness, at what age did it begin? _____ years old

On an average day, how much are you bothered by the 8 symptoms listed below? (Rate each symptom from 0 to 10, where 10 is the worst it could be, and where 0 means you have none of that symptom)

Dizziness = ___ /10
Nausea = ___ /10
Anxiety = ___ /10
Headache = ___ /10
Neckache = ___ /10
Unsteady with walking = ___ /10
Sensitivity to light = ___ /10
Difficulty reading = ___ /10

Please record any additional symptoms you may be experiencing or specific concerns that you have about your eyes / vision:

_____
_____
_____
_____
_____
_____

©2013 Vision Specialists of Michigan

259

How To Score The Pediatric VHSQ

The Pediatric Vertical Heterophoria Symptom Questionnaire (P-VHSQ) has been designed to detect those patients 17 years old and younger whose headache, dizziness, anxiety or neck ache might be due to a visually mediated cause (usually Vertical Heterophoria). Feel free to make a copy of the questionnaire and use it yourself, or give it to a friend or loved one you suspect might have VH. Scoring is performed by summing the values given to Questions 1 – 27 as follows:

Always = 3

Frequently = 2

Occasionally = 1

Never = 0

If the score is $\geq$ 15, consultation with a Neurovisual optometrist is recommended.

Pediatric Vertical Heterophoria Symptom Questionnaire (P-VHSQ)

for children 17 years old and younger

Vision Specialists of Michigan

2550 S. Telegraph Road, Suite 100   Bloomfield Hills, Michigan 48302   (248) 258-9000
www.VSofM.com   Fax (248) 499-6372

Name: _____   Email: _____   Date: _____

Best phone number: _____   Back-up phone number: _____

Directions: Children - answer these questions together with your Parents. For every question, check the answer that best describes your situation. If you wear glasses or contact lenses, answer the questions assuming that you are wearing them. Please answer every question.

Never = Never
Occasionally = Less than 1 time / week
Frequently = At least 1 time / week
Always = Everyday

	NEVER	OCCASIONALLY	FREQUENTLY	ALWAYS
1. Do you have headaches or face pain?				
2. Do your eyes hurt and/or does it hurt to move your eyes?				
3. Do you have neck pain or a stiff neck or upper back pain?				
4. Do you have stomach aches or nausea?				

5. Do you get car sickness or motion sickness?

6. Did you get sick in the car seat when you were a small child?

7. Do you get sick to your stomach or nauseous on swings or circular rides?

8. Does riding in the car give you headaches or stomach aches?

9. Do you have trouble reading in the car?

10. Do you feel clumsy or klutzy or uncoordinated?

11. When you are walking, do you bump into people or furniture or door frames?

12. Do you feel funny or dizzy when you bend over and stand back up quickly?

13. Are you anxious or nervous?

14. In grocery stores or malls, do you stay close (cling) to your Mom or Dad? (Do you feel uncomfortable in grocery stores or malls?)

15. Do you tend to play alone or with just a few other kids? (Do you tend to play apart from the main group of kids?)

16. Is reading hard for you or are you a slow reader?

17. Do you have to read the same thing a couple of times to really understand it?

NEVER	OCCASIONALLY	FREQUENTLY	ALWAYS						

18. Do you use your finger or a ruler or a piece of paper to help you keep your place when you are reading?

19. Do you skip lines or lose your place when you are reading?

20. When you read, does it look like the letters are moving OR does it seem like words are bumping into each other?

21. Do bright lights hurt your eyes?

22. Do you close or cover one eye to make it easier to see?

23. Do you have trouble catching baseballs or footballs or Frisbees?

24. Do you ever see two of everything (double vision)?

25. Is it hard for you to watch 3-D movies?

26. When reading or working on the computer, do your eyes feel tired or does your vision get blurry?

27. When looking at the blackboard at school, do your eyes feel tired or does your vision get blurry?

Mom / Dad: Has your child ever been diagnosed with:

Learning disability (LD)? ☐ YES ☐ NO	Reading disability?	☐ YES ☐ NO
Dyslexia? ☐ YES ☐ NO	ADD / ADHD?	☐ YES ☐ NO
Torticollis? ☐ YES ☐ NO	Migraines or headache disorder?	☐ YES ☐ NO
Lazy eye? ☐ YES ☐ NO	Traumatic brain injury or concussion?	☐ YES ☐ NO

Does your child blink their eyes a lot / much more then most children? ☐ YES ☐ NO

Are your child's verbal skills far ahead of their reading skills? ☐ YES ☐ NO

Has your child ever had an eye operation? ☐ YES ☐ NO

On an average day, how much are you bothered by the 8 symptoms listed below? (Rate each symptom from 0 to 10, where 10 is the worst it could be, and where 0 means you have none of that symptom)	Please record any additional symptoms you may be experiencing, or specific concerns that you have about your eyes / vision:
Dizziness = ___ / 10	
Nausea = ___ / 10	
Anxiety = ___ / 10	
Headache = ___ / 10	
Neckache = ___ / 10	
Unsteady with walking= ___ / 10	
Sensitivity to light = ___ / 10	
Reading difficulty = ___ / 10	

APPENDIX C

What is Vertical Heterophoria?

A DESCRIPTION FOR EVERYONE

Vertical Heterophoria (VH) is an uncommonly recognized and poorly understood visual condition where the two eyes have difficulty looking directly at the image being viewed. They are slightly out of alignment vertically, which can lead to double vision. The brain prevents the impending double vision by using the eye muscles to correct the misalignment and keep both eyes pointing directly at the image. However, using the eye muscles in this manner over a long period of time overworks them, causing them to become strained and fatigued, which precipitates the symptoms of VH.

Strained eye muscles cause headaches, usually in the front of the face or in the temples. As the muscles strain, they become fatigued and they quiver, causing the eyes to move rapidly but minutely, which creates the feeling of dizziness, lightheadedness, disorientation and a sense of imbalance. Those who suffer from VH may also have other symptoms in addition to those of headaches and dizziness. These include:

- additional **pain symptoms** such as face ache, eye pain or pain with eye movement (symptoms similar to sinus problems, migraines, TMJ problems); neck ache and upper back pain due to a head tilt (symptoms similar to spinal misalignment problems);

- additional **vestibular symptoms** such as motion sickness, nausea, poor depth perception, unsteadiness while walking or drifting to one side while walking ("I've always been clumsy"), lack of coordination (symptoms are similar to those seen in patients with MS, sequela of a stroke, an inner ear disorder or Meniere's Disease);

- **reading symptoms** such as difficulty with concentration (symptoms are similar to those experienced with ADHD), difficulty with reading and comprehension, skipping lines while reading, losing one's place while reading, words running together while reading (symptoms similar to those seen with a learning disability);

- **vision symptoms** such as blurred vision, double or overlapping vision, shadowed vision (symptoms similar to those seen in patients with MS); light sensitivity, difficulty with glare or reflection;

- **psychological symptoms** such as feeling overwhelmed or anxious when in large contained spaces like malls or big box stores, feeling overwhelmed or anxious in crowds (symptoms similar to those seen in patients with anxiety or agoraphobia).

This condition may be caused by head trauma / traumatic brain injury (TBI), stroke, or neurological disorders. However, most often this is a condition you are born with (i.e. - one eye is higher than the other eye; eye muscle or nerve abnormalities). It may take years before symptoms occur, as the body will do the best it can to try and compensate for these problems.

The severity and number of symptoms vary from person to person – some people are much more affected than others.

268

This condition tends to run in families.

To correct this problem, the optometrist adds prism to your lenses. Prism is a way of making the lenses such that the image seen by the eye is moved up or down or to the side – whatever is needed to allow the eyes to point in the correct direction without straining the eye muscles. Proper prism correction leads to a reduction of symptoms of (on average) about 80%.

Pathophysiology of Vertical Heterophoria
A DESCRIPTION FOR THE MEDICAL PROFESSIONAL

Vertical heterophoria is a form of binocular vision dysfunction where there appears to be a faulty alignment message from the brain that causes the phoric posture (line of sight) of one eye to be higher than that of the other eye and to be vertically crossed (*vertical transphoria* - Figure 1 – dotted lines pointing to FP). To avoid diplopia, two physiological mechanisms are employed:

1. The eyes undergo *compensatory vertical divergence*, moving the lines-of-sight / phoric posture back to midline (solid lines pointing to T – Figure 2). The conflict between the faulty message (causing vertical transphoria) and the compensatory message (causing compensatory vertical divergence) results in overuse of the opposing elevator and depressor extraocular muscles (EOM's), causing EOM strain and fatigue, which leads to headache, dizziness and anxiety.

2. Tilting the head toward the shoulder vertically realigns the images, but this leads to neck ache [Figures 4-5].

How is VH treated?

Vertically realigning prismatic lenses are used to move the image vertically so that the image strikes the fovia while the eyes are in their baseline phoric posture / line if sight (where no EOM strain is occurring) [Figure 3].

Why is there so little VH research?

VH has been an uncommonly diagnosed and poorly understood disorder. We suspect that this is due in large part to the inconsistent performance of the current tests used to identify the direction and amount of VH which makes diagnosing, treating and researching this condition almost impossible.

How do we diagnose VH?

We developed an alternative method for diagnosing and treating VH that does not rely upon the use of the current tests. In those patients with physical findings or symptoms suggestive of VH, we utilize the Vertical Heterophoria Symptom Questionnaire (VHSQ - a validated VH symptom assessment instrument developed by the authors to determine VH symptom burden) to identify those who would benefit from binocular vision subspecialist consultation (*VH suspects*). During the consultation it is ascertained whether appropriately applied vertically correcting prismatic lenses result in significant symptom reduction within a short time frame (20-30 minutes) (*Prism Challenge*). Those who have significant symptom reduction with Prism Challenge are diagnosed with VH.

Figure 1:

Phoric Position of the Eyes in Vertical Transphoria (newly described phoric position)

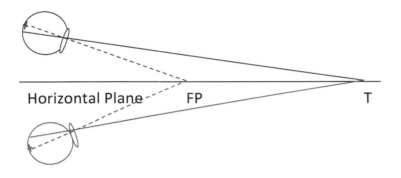

(For ease of demonstration, this Figure is showing eye position as if the head is tilted, with the left eye high.)

The lines of sight (phoric position) of the eyes (dotted lines pointing to FP) are vertically misaligned – they are crossed or *Transphoric*. Note that the target image (solid line) misses the fovea. This will cause blurred vision or vertical diplopia if not corrected.

Figure 2:

Compensatory Vertical Divergence (newly described eye movement)

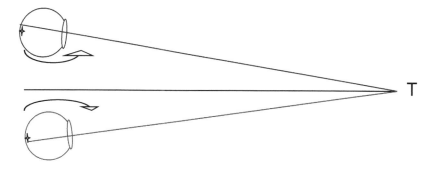

This eye movement (arrows) compensates for Vertical Transphoria by elevating the higher eye and depressing the lower eye utilizing the opposing elevator and depressor muscles. This effectively brings the target image to the foveas. However, this creates increased stress and tension in the initial elevator and depressor muscles as well as the opposing compensatory elevator and depressor muscles.

Figure 3:

Prismatic Correction of Compensatory Vertical Divergence

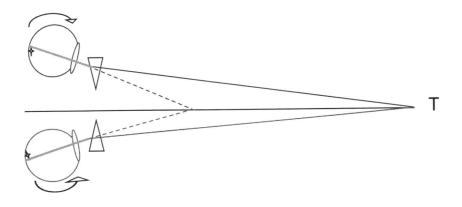

Vertical prismatic lenses align the Image from Target (solid line) with Line of Sight (dotted line), allowing the image to strike the fovea while the eyes are in their transphoric posture. This allows elimination of the use of the opposing compensatory elevator and depressor muscles, eliminating the need for Compensatory Vertical Divergence (arrows). This eliminates the extraocular muscle strain and fatigue, and concomitantly alleviates the symptoms of VH.

Figure 4: Head Tilt

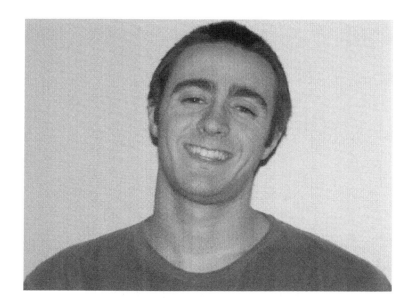

Figure 5:

Effects of Head Tilt on the Projection of an Image onto the Retina in Vertical Heterophoria

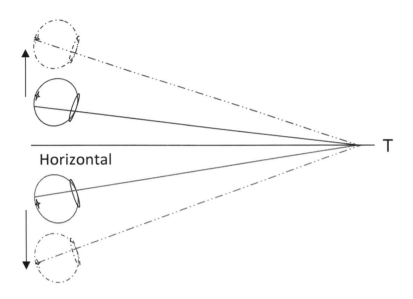

Horizontal

T

Tilting the head increases the vertical separation of the eyes (ghosted images), which brings the Target Image closer to the foveas.

Index (by Symptoms)

(Cited by Story number)

N

nausea (also see *weight loss*), 2, 7, 11, 12, 15, 17, 18, 19, 21, 22,
    26, 32, 34, 40

neck and shoulder pain / tension, 2, 7, 14, 16, 21, 23, 25, 29, 35,
    38

O

off-balanced walking – see *walking problems*

overwhelmed in crowds – see *anxiety*

overwhelmed in large spaces – see *anxiety*

P

panic attacks – see *anxiety*

pediatric – see *children*

peripheral vision difficulty – see *vision problems*

R

reading problems, 5, 7, 8, 11, 12, 17, 18, 20, 21, 22, 25, 26
    difficulty with reading comprehension, 6, 14, 39
    dyslexia, 37
    loses place while reading, 2, 13
    reading fatigue, 39
    skips lines while reading, 22
    visual hallucination of letters / words moving, 6, 17

ringing in ears – see *ear ringing*

S

sensitivity to light – see *light sensitivity*

sensitivity to sound – see *sound sensitivity*

shadowed images – see *vision problems*

shoulder pain / tension – see *neck pain / tension*

skipping lines while reading – see *reading problems*

sound sensitivity, 9, 30, 34

spinning – see *vertigo*

squint, 20

suicidal ideation, 1, 28

sweating, 11

T

traumatic brain injury (TBI), 1, 2, 3, 4, 6, 7, 8, 9, 10, 11, 12, 13, 14, 15

    TBI, military acquired, 5, 15,

teenager – see *children*

tinnitus – see *ear ringing*

U

unclear vision – see *vision problems*

upper back pain/ tension – see *neck pain / tension*

V

veering while walking – see *walking problems*

vertigo, 10, 22, 24, 27, 31, 32, 34, 35

vision problems

    blurred vision (near or far), 3, 4, 13, 14, 15, 22, 25

    closing / covering an eye to improve visual clarity, 23

    decreased visual acuity, 8

    difficulty being fit with glasses, 27

    difficulty with peripheral vision, 27, 29

    double vision / diplopia, 3, 8, 14, 17, 18, 36

    shadowed vision, 6, 20

    visual hallucination of letters / words moving – see *reading problems*

W

walking problems,

    drifting / veering while walking, 13, 16, 17, 18, 19, 20, 21, 23, 34, 37

    disequilibrium, 5

    unbalanced or unsteady gait / walking, 1, 7, 8, 12, 28, 36

weight loss (also see *nausea*), 2, 26

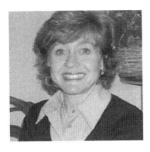

Dr. Debby Feinberg is Director of Vision Specialists of Michigan, where she has been performing pioneering work on Vertical Heterophoria since 1995. She and her colleagues have successfully treated over 7000 patients locally, nationally and internationally utilizing realigning prismatic eyeglass lenses. She resides in Commerce Township, Michigan, is the mother of two wonderful boys, and is married to Dr. Mark Rosner.

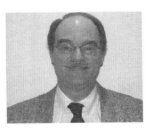

Dr. Mark Rosner is Director of Research at Vision Specialists Institute, the research and teaching arm of Vision Specialists of Michigan. He has been the main writer on all of the academic papers and posters. He and Dr. Feinberg and other members of the research team have presented this information at local, national and international conferences. He is a practicing Emergency Physician, and is married to Dr. Debby Feinberg.

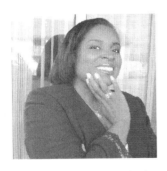

Sherry Brantley is the author of several books including: *"Choices—The Power is Within You,"* and *"Seven Successful Strategies for Divorced Parents."* She is an Inspirational Speaker and a CLC (Certified Life Coach) specializing in Goal-Setting, with a concentrated focus on completing the all-important steps to attaining goals. Sherry's next project includes *'Sweet Potato Pie for the Heart,'* a compilation of true, personal stories submitted by people who have had unique, uplifting experiences that have been life-changing for them in some way.

Made in the USA
Charleston, SC
27 February 2013